The
Foundation of the Chronic Miasms

The Foundation of the Chronic Miasms *in the* Practice of Homeopathy

Henny Heudens–Mast

Edited by
M. Teresa Bland, CCH
with Louise Divine

SIMILIA PRESS

Similia Press
8470 Caraway Court
Orlando, Florida 32819
USA
www.similiapress.com

First Edition
Third Printing

Compilation and First Edit: Mary A. Junewick
Editing and Proofreading: Donna Cay Tharpe, Extreme Editing
Book Cover Design: Valerie MacLeod, Sir Speedy Printing
Cover Image: *Nova Party* 1998, by Terry Wright
Composition: William H. Brunson Typography Services
Indexing: Lydia A. Junewick, MLS

ISBN 0-9773057-0-8 Hardcover
ISBN 0-9773057-1-6 Softcover

For all homeopaths who wish to follow in the footsteps of the old masters to further develop their understanding of the chronic miasms, and to all homeopaths who experience the deep joy of working with the healing possibilities of the human organism, I do hope that the information in this book, which is drawn from my experience in practicing this very important part of our science, will better equip you to treat and cure our patients of their complicated health problems.

Henny Heudens-Mast
Leuven, Belgium 2005

Fractal—"Nova Party" by Terry Wright

A "nova" occurs when a star suddenly becomes intensely brighter and then gradually returns to its original brightness over a period of weeks to years. Stars "go nova" when they eject some of their material in the form of a cloud and thus become more luminous and brilliant for a time.

Fractals are images derived from mathematical formulas and generated by computer software. A fractal is a geometric shape repeated at ever-smaller scales. Therefore, fractals are self-similar and infinite—that is one can (in theory) zoom forever into a fractal and continue to see permutations of the same shapes and forms.

For information on Fractals or image designer Terry Wright
visit www.eclectasy.com

Similia Press
8470 Caraway Court
Orlando, Florida 32819
USA
www.similiapress.com

CONTENTS

Foreword xi
Editors' Preface xiii
Acknowedgments xv

Introduction The Foundation of the Chronic Miasms in the Practice of Homeopathy 1
What Is a Miasm? 1
Can We Cure the Psoric Miasm? 3
Psora, Active and Latent 4
Latent Psora Awakened 4
Energetic Reactions and Suppression 5
Multiple Miasms 7
Symptoms as a Guide to the Miasms 9
Miasmatic Prescribing and Long-Term Case Management 10
All Homeopathic Treatment Addresses Miasms 12

Chapter 1 Psora and the Psoric Miasm 13
Mental and Emotional Symptoms and Expressions of the Psoric Miasm 13
General and Physical Symptoms and Modalities of the Psoric Miasm 20
The Psoric Miasm in Infants and Children 25
Psoric Remedies 28
Psora Case 1: Boy With Cough and Delayed Growth 29
Psora Case 2: Boy With Encopresis and Behavior Problems 42

Chapter 2 Syphilis and the Syphilitic Miasm 53
Mental and Emotional Symptoms and Expressions of the Syphilitic Miasm 54
Professions and Behaviors 58
General and Physical Symptoms and Modalities of the Syphilitic Miasm 65
The Syphilitic Miasm in Infants and Children 72
Miasms in Pregnancy 75

Syphilitic Remedies 75
Syphilis Case 1: Baby Girl With Reflux and Thrush 76
Syphilis Case 2: Six-Year-Old Boy With Pervasive Developmental Delay 84
Prescribe Only When Necessary 106
Apply the Miasms 107

Chapter 3 Sycosis and the Sycotic Miasm 109
Mental and Emotional Symptoms and Expressions of the Sycotic Miasm 110
General and Physical Symptoms and Modalities of the Sycotic Miasm 118
The Sycotic Miasm in Infants and Children 122
Sycotic Remedies 123
Sycosis Case 1: Man With Nephrotic Syndrome 124
Sycosis Case 2: Boy With Recurrent Throat Infections 134

Chapter 4 Tuberculosis and the Tubercular Miasm 143
Mental and Emotional Symptoms and Expressions of the Tubercular Miasm 149
General and Physical Symptoms and Modalities of the Tubercular Miasm 153
The Tubercular Miasm in Infants and Children 155
Tubercular Remedies 156
Tubercular Case 1: Girl With Allergies, Convulsions, and Tantrums 158
Tubercular Case 2: Man With Prostatitis 169

Chapter 5 Cancer and the Cancer Miasm 181
Cancer Miasm vs. Cancer Disease 184
Mental and Emotional Symptoms and Expressions of the Cancer Miasm 186
General and Physical Symptoms of the Cancer Miasm 189
Cancer Remedies 190
Treating the Disease of Cancer 192
Homeopathy at the End of Life 195
Cancer Case 1: Woman With Marriage Problems, Depression, and Anger 196

Chapter 6 Other Miasms Emerging 205
Using Knowledge of the Miasms 207
Miasms Seen Metaphorically 208
Case 1: Man With AIDS 208

Chapter 7 One Diagnosis, Three Disease States 215
Case 1: First Woman With MS 215
Case 2: Second Woman With MS 219
Case 3: Third Woman With MS 224
Concluding Remarks on MS Cases 229

Chapter 8 Conclusion 231
Getting to the "Basis" of Disease 232
The Progression of Miasms 233
Recognizing SRP Symptoms and the Miasm Needing Treatment 234
The Path to Cure 235
What Influences Your Miasmatic Prescriptions? 237
Fearless Perseverance 237

Appendices 239
Appendix 1: Comparative Summary of the Chronic Miasms 239
Appendix 2: Comparative Chart—Miasmatic Tendencies and Expressions 244

Index 247

FOREWORD

Henny Heudens-Mast is well known to European homeopaths as a brilliant contemporary interpreter of classical principles. Fluent in four languages, she has taught for decades in her own school in Belgium and in seminars throughout Europe and Scandinavia. Until now, North America has had relatively little opportunity to learn from Henny, as she teaches here only twice a year. This book marks Henny's first widespread outreach to the American homeopathic community.

Readers who are new to Henny should be warned: she offers no quick fixes or shortcuts. There is nothing faddish, nothing showy, about her teaching: for Henny, homeopathy is a lifelong pursuit demanding continuous study and offering continuous rewards. Casual readers may miss the depth of her message because her approach is so methodical and pragmatic. Those who read carefully and, even more importantly, put her ideas to the test of use will find a treasure trove here.

One crucial ingredient in Henny's teaching is her modern application of classical principles. Observing her own 30-year practice from the perspective she gains from masters such as Hahnemann, Hering, and Kent, she has recognized the contemporary face of the disease processes they described. The same miasms, she asserts, are still evident in today's population, although they may look different because they are further evolved and their image is refracted through a different cultural and temporal lens. Providing concrete examples, Henny teaches how to discern the chronic miasms in our modern context.

Perhaps the most significant aspect of Henny's approach to the chronic miasms is the window it provides into the nature of disease. Hahnemann writes in Aphorism 3 that the homeopath must know diseases, medicines, and the application of the one to the other. Significantly, he names diseases first, suggesting that the foundation of our work is a clear understanding of the nature and dynamics of disease. Indeed, it is our knowledge of the true basis of disease and hence our insight into the process of cure that sets homeopathy apart from all other modalities. Yet, because so much of our contemporary discussion focuses on Hahnemann's second and third points, we run the risk of losing touch with the very foundation of homeopathy.

Through Henny, miasmatic philosophy becomes neither simply a static classification system nor just another clinical tool, but rather a method of understanding and influencing the dynamic processes of health and disease.

Applied miasmatic philosophy can transform homeopathic practice. It creates a larger totality in case analysis; it makes sense of seemingly unrelated symptoms; it has predictive value for the processes of both disease and cure; it facilitates long-term case management; and it opens the door for the use of lesser known remedies by virtue of their relation to the miasmatic picture. As this book's chapter on a possible emerging AIDS miasm reflects, understanding the dynamics of miasms also allows us to recognize and treat new miasms.

Like her intellectual forebear Samuel Hahnemann, Henny bases her teaching on objective observation in a clinical setting. In this empirical method, theory comes directly from experience. A book can only begin to open the student to this approach: like a driver's manual, it explains the rules, but it is no substitute for demonstration and hands-on learning. Henny's seminars, with live cases and live followup over many years, offer the opportunity to apply the information in this book. Readers who find this book compelling should be encouraged to learn more by studying with its author and putting her method to the ultimate test, experience.

Ann Jerome, PhD, CCH
Director, Academy of Classical Homeopathy

EDITORS' PREFACE

In 1994, when Henny Heudens-Mast first came to teach in the U.S., no one was talking about the importance of "miasms"—no one was teaching from a miasmatic perspective and surely no one knew the depth of what Henny meant to spark in each of her students when she went to her white board and drew pictures of three different types of warts, each classifiable by its miasmatic characteristics. So innocent, she turned to her class, saw their eyes wide in excited amazement, and asked, "This is interesting to you?"

To some in that class what Henny had said about miasms was not interesting. To some it was the single most influential day in their homeopathic study to date, a light offering a clearer and more complete understanding of the nature of disease and the power of the individual vital force to express itself. And they could not shake loose of Henny, or her tenacious pursuit of Hahnemann's Paragraph 2, "... rapid, gentle and permanent restoration of health according to clearly realizable principles." The journey had begun.

Our original purpose for setting these ideas to paper was simple. We thought to provide a basic context in which newcomers to the miasms, to miasmatic understanding and case management could begin their study. A pamphlet perhaps, a basic outline which would give any who chose to attend one of Henny's seminars enough understanding of miasms that they would not be lost when she got to the part in case analysis where she again lifted her pen to the white board and began her diagrammatic classification of each symptom according to its miasmatic influence within the patient; when she asked the class to differentiate each possible remedy miasmatically; when she asked students to support their prescription decision – why a remedy from this miasm now, and what to expect from this prescription. And the journey continues.

We invite you to think of this book as a seminar. We have compiled information from Henny's international classes and seminars, given from 1996 to 2004, to create a sort of narrative encyclopedia of her teachings on the chronic miasms. We have organized this material as Henny often organizes a week-long seminar, beginning from principles and proceeding to concrete information, with increasingly detailed illustrations as the week goes on.

As a written record of oral teaching, this book retains many characteristics of the spoken word. You can expect some repetition for reinforcement of key points and some fruitful tangents here and there. You will find spontaneous analogies, anecdotes, and clinical advice mixed in with the planned structure. Henny sometimes refers specifically to particular works, but more often, references to the old masters are embedded in her thought. You may hear Hahnemann, Hering, and Kent speaking through her.

Henny explains in the Introduction that in her taxonomy, every remedy and every patient contain elements of more than one miasm. For simplicity's sake, she speaks of "a psoric remedy" or "a syphilitic case" rather than "a primarily psoric remedy" or "a mostly syphilitic case," and we have retained this habit in hopes that the reader can hold on to her true meaning while enjoying the economy of words.

We have compiled her primary information on miasms and miasmatic prescribing as a foundation for further understanding and practice. Henny has two other books that are being translated from German, which further illustrate and apply her homeopathic understanding. These books, one dealing with Hysteria and the other with ADHD, will be in print in English in the near future.

Sadly, some of what Henny offers through her teaching cannot be captured in book form. Though we have done our best to include the depth of information presented in seminar settings, we encourage you to seek out her seminars to experience the full range of what she offers her "colleagues," as she respectfully addresses her students. One significant example is her consummate professional ethics, which she models in her case-based seminars. Patients whose cases are presented here have given permission, and identifying details have been changed to protect their privacy.

Along with its information, this book's tone, logic, humor, and much of the language are uniquely Henny's. We hope that some of her personality, her compassionate objectivity, her wit, and her profound common sense shine through these pages.

M. Teresa Bland
Louise Divine
Lutea Press, LLC

ACKNOWLEDGMENTS

We would like to express our deep appreciation and gratitude to the following people, all who have selflessly given their time, energy and talents without measure to bring the voice of Henny in homeopathy to the pages of a book.

Holly Lacy, CCH, angel abundance of the universe, for her diligent and bodacious skills both in homeopathic understanding and in seminar transcription, for her friendship, and for her generosity of spirit.

Mary A. Junewick, editor and homeopath, whose enthusiasm and respect for Henny's work, knowledge of editing and publishing, initial compilation and professional advice gave us structure and inspiration from which we could both launch and complete this project.

Donna Cay Tharpe, editor extreme, talent abounding, for her unfailing eye, her word sense, her activism and her unflagging dedication to the vision, not to mention the hundred or so read-throughs even when she did not have the time. No words can really thank.

Katie Alexander Hunter, our heartfelt thanks for her generous support and deep commitment to homeopathy. She recognized early on the importance of Henny's teaching for the serious homeopathic student.

Ann Jerome, PhD, CCH, teacher and rescue artist, for sharing her writing talent and her deep understanding of homeopathy, and for her diplomacy, guidance and keen intelligence.

Bill Brunson, for his professional standards, for his patience, and for his ability to make us feel as though we were not the fledglings that we know we are.

Karen Cohen, DC, CCH, Julia A. Eastman, DOM, CCH and **Tina Torri, ND, LAc**, for their time and their invaluable suggestions, and most of all, for their collegial spirit.

Paul Herscu, ND, for introducing us to Henny Heudens-Mast.

And to all of Henny's patients who had the courage to give their cases in front of so many, and from whom we learned so much, we are most surely grateful.

INTRODUCTION

THE FOUNDATION OF THE CHRONIC MIASMS IN THE PRACTICE OF HOMEOPATHY

What is the highest goal that we all share as homeopaths? We all know the answer. It is the tenet on which we begin and end every prescription; it is the charge with which Hahnemann began his teaching to us. Our goal is GENTLE, RAPID, and PERMANENT restoration of health in our patients "according to clearly comprehensible principles." How many of our prescriptions are actually able to accomplish this goal? Our choices of remedies for our patients may perform gently and our patients' responses may be rapid, but how often do we know for certain that our patients are permanently restored to health?

This is the very problem that Hahnemann faced in his own practice almost 200 years ago and the challenge that ultimately led him to understand the nature of disease in the larger context of miasms.

What Is a Miasm?

Even when Hahnemann had established the homeopathic law of cure and was applying it in his practice, even when he knew how powerful homeopathy is, his meticulous and open-minded observation of his patients showed him a problem. Many patients responded well to a remedy initially and felt better for a time, even to a point of symptom-free health, yet later relapsed and returned with the same complaint, sometimes increased in its troubling nature. We know from reading Hahnemann's *Chronic Diseases* that he devoted 12 years (1816–1828) trying to fully understand why this could happen. He knew that the remedies themselves were working, so he looked more deeply into the true nature of the diseases.

In *Chronic Diseases*, Hahnemann tells us that his experience in practice confirmed that the non-venereal chronic illnesses, though treated correctly homeopathically, always returned in some new form, often with new symptoms or increased complaints. The new symptoms, which appeared after homeopathic treatment, were his clue to the existence of a deeper and more pervasive disease. Where he had thought that he was seeing and treating the whole disease, he now understood that these supposedly isolated illnesses were only fragments of a deeper original chronic disease, and that in order to bring permanent cure, his remedies had to address the original disease as a whole.

This is the meaning of chronic disease, miasmatic disease: a deeper disease that rules at the very foundation of the energy and well-being of a person with ever changing and ever increasing symptoms unless treated "artfully" homeopathically. These changes, in the form of new symptoms, are the voice of the underlying original chronic miasmatic disease and must be treated with the understanding that they are forming a picture, not of a separate "well-defined" disease, but of the original disease itself. Unless these chronic patterns and influences are addressed, the disease will go on progressing until death.

Miasms are the basis of all disease. Miasms can be inherited or acquired from contagion or suppression. The only way to truly cure our patients is by addressing the miasms.

In studying the miasms, our goal is to learn to recognize and understand these chronic disease patterns as they manifest in our patients and in the remedies we use to treat them. With this understanding, we can help our patients reach the highest level of health. Without this understanding, our practice of homeopathy can suffer "relapse."

Miasms are named for particular illnesses from which they originate, but due to their further development, miasms are much more far-reaching within the organism than the illness that started them. As a seed spreads a root system far into the surrounding soil, so does the illness establish the miasm that extends, complicates, and perpetuates its influence.

Hahnemann teaches that psora, from the "itch," is the basis of all disease and hence of all other miasms as well, perhaps dating back to the beginning of human existence. Since psora is contracted by mere touch, its spread throughout all of humanity was unavoidable. There is no choice involved; one only has to touch or shake hands with a psoric person to get psora. Hahnemann taught that everyone had psora and that, even without the visible presence of skin eruptions or known history of symptoms of the original itch disease, almost everyone could expect to have some kind of secondary symptoms of the internal psoric disease such as fear, coldness, or burning.

Can We Cure the Psoric Miasm?

Our goal, we know, is GENTLE, RAPID, and PERMANENT restoration of health in our patients. This was Hahnemann's passion and our charge. He tells us that without artfully correct homeopathic treatment there is no hope of curing the original psoric disease. During his time, he saw that in patients whose psora was not fully developed internally, he and some of his colleagues had great success with the medicines that were fully proved at the time. He also recognized the difficulty in finding the same success in cases where the patients' psora was fully developed, especially where it was complicated by other miasms as well. Of course, our goal of curing psora is the same as was Hahnemann's, but in my experience of over 30 years treating our modern population, I have not seen the basic psoric disease completely eradicated in my patients.

What are some of the differences between Hahnemann's patients and ours? We live in a very different world. We breathe different air, eat different food and drink different water. Our patients live under the influence of vaccination, synthetic chemicals, artificial ingredients, genetically altered foods, and pervasive suppression of illness, both in these individuals and in their forebears. The generations between Hahnemann's time and ours have produced a weaker and more miasmatically complicated population.

In Hahnemann's time, some people had only psora, and even then he saw the great suffering that this chronic disease caused and how difficult it was to truly cure. Today, it would be very difficult to find children born with psora only, for it would mean that their parents, grandparents, great-grandparents, and earlier ancestors for generations also had only psora. This would indeed be a very rare occurrence.

Hahnemann set the highest goal, and we must still work toward it. Like Hahnemann, we must also be aware of the particular nature of our own patients in our own time and of the changes occurring within the disease state of these patients. One thing this involves is recognizing the difference between an active and a latent miasm.

Psora, Active and Latent

Psora is with us; it is part of humankind. It can be active or it can be latent. Active psora causes symptoms. When we treat a patient whose active psora calms down, he then feels fine. Psora then becomes a sleeping, latent psora, and perhaps that latent psora will remain sleeping for a long time. As long as our patients remain in a latent psoric state, they feel well.

In my experience, latent psora is the best possible situation for all patients. Everyone has minor physical complaints; no one is perfect. If we could live forever, in perfect bodies, we would know that psora had been cured. As long as we have imperfect bodies and die, we know we have psora in our "rucksack." As long as psora stays there, sleeping, it will not cause great disturbances and will not keep us in a state of illness. However, sleeping psora is apt to be awakened by certain influences and experiences. Recognizing when this happens is one key to successful case management in the long run.

Latent Psora Awakened

Here is a good example of how latency works. Let's say that I am feeling fine. I have a good situation and no serious problems, but I have latent psora. One day, somebody comes to tell me, "Your homeopathic clinic caught fire and has totally burned down. Two patients died in the fire." I have the psoric miasm, so what can happen to me? I may feel anxiety. I may feel faint or chilly. My knees may give out, and I may fall to the ground. Or I may feel paralyzed and unable to do anything. All of these would be normal reactions. If I am quite healthy, these reactions will go away by themselves, despite my latent psora. But because there is latent psora, there is also the possibility that my reactions of that moment will stay, creating a state in which problems continue to develop and I am unable to recover my former energy. From my latent psoric state, where I felt fine, I am now in active psora, where I can develop any number of possible conditions, depending on my unique predispositions. Perhaps delusions or mania, perhaps melancholy, perhaps weeping and fear to be alone, perhaps chronic headaches or fatigue and trembling or unexplained muscle pain and stiffness, perhaps paralysis or multiple sclerosis—any problem that is already within my predisposition can develop. These disparate conditions might not seem to be related to the shock that awakened my psora, but they most definitely are. We can trace their interrelationship through their shared connection to the miasm.

Successful homeopathic treatment renders the miasms latent. Stressors to which the individual is sensitive can subsequently reawaken them.

One of the characteristics of psora is sensitivity to repeated fearful situations. We will discuss characteristics of psora in more depth, but for now you can see in this example that because I am Ms. Psora and I am predisposed to ailments from fear, this message could trigger in me an active psoric state. At that moment of shock, or even many years later, I would need a psoric remedy. In our clinics, many patients say, "Since I suffered this or that, my health has declined." They experience flare-ups of their latent state, or their latent state is awakened or becomes active. From the character of the symptoms, we can discern which miasm(s) has(ve) been awakened. When there is a trigger of anxiety, fear, or bad news and if many complaints have developed since that first moment of shock, it is probably a sign of the psoric miasm.

Energetic Reactions and Suppression

If everyone has psora, why does a shock push some people into a chronic state, while others have a reaction that may last only minutes or days? One contributing factor is the individual energy level available for counter-reaction and healing. Another is suppression of the symptoms that occur after the shock.

Suppression complicates the case and causes the miasm to develop further, so that more serious symptoms may ensue.

Shock or stress to the organism causes a reaction on the part of the vital force in an effort to correct the imbalance. If the vital energy of the patient is strong enough to overcome the stress on its own, it will do so. We have all seen it happen. It may require increased rest and an hour or two or a day or two of symptoms, perhaps diarrhea, as an outlet for the internal stress created by the shock, but if I am healthy enough and have healthy high energy, my vital force can bring my organism back into balance, back into my latent psoric state, without need of a remedy. If my energy is less or the shock is too great, I may need a homeopathic remedy. Now my energy will improve; the diarrhea can go on for as long as the stressed system needs an outlet, and when balance is reached, my organism will cure the diarrhea.

If, however, I receive a shock, get diarrhea, and take a medicine to stop the diarrhea, the outlet for the stress of my shocking experience is suppressed, and the stress will go somewhere else in the organism because I have blocked the natural action of the vital force. Any intervention that is targeted to eliminate the particular symptom can have this effect. As homeopaths, we must always remember what we know to be the laws of health and disease.

Suppression can be accomplished by homeopathic prescribing that is too narrow, as well as by allopathic medication or any other suppressive intervention.

If we could measure our energy levels on a scale from 10 to 95 percent, we might better predict how our bodies would react to stress. When we have high energy—say 95 percent—and we are psoric, our bodies will react strongly. Perhaps we will get diarrhea or faint—problems that are quickly finished. But if our vital energy is lower, if there is a history of suppression as with the majority of today's patient population, or if we are under constant stress from poor nutrition, bad air, etc., then we are more likely to respond with more serious and more chronic pathology.

Here are a few of the more than 600 rubrics in *The Complete Repertory, Millennium Edition,* that confirm suppression of one symptom producing another. Numbers in parentheses indicate the number of remedies in the specific rubric:

MIND; AILMENTS from; anger, *vexation; suppressed* (23)
MIND; HYSTERIA; *menses; scanty or suppressed* (16)
MIND; ERUPTIONS or hemorrhoids; *mental symptoms agg. after suppressed* (27)

NOSE; EPISTAXIS; *general; menses; suppressed* (24)
HEAD PAIN; GENERAL; *coryza; with; suppressed* (19)
HEAD PAIN; GENERAL; *eruptions, after suppressed* (9)
RESPIRATION; ASTHMATIC; *eruptions; suppressed, after* (20)
COUGH; ERUPTIONS; *from suppressed* (5)
CHEST; HEMORRHAGE; *hemorrhoidal flow, after suppression of* (9)
CHEST; PHTHISIS pulmonalis; *diarrhea, from suppressed* (1)
CHEST; PAIN; *rheumatic; heart, endocarditis lenta; suppressed, from* (7)
CHEST; PAIN; *sore, heart; perspiration of foot, agg., from suppressed* (2)
EXTREMITIES; PARALYSIS; general; *suppressed; eruptions* (5)
EXTREMITY PAIN; GENERAL; *rheumatic; diarrhea; checked, suppressed, from* (2)
EXTREMITY PAIN; RHEUMATIC; *gonorrhea, after suppressed* (31)
SLEEP; SLEEPLESSNESS; *suppressed secretion, from* (1)
GENERALS; CONVULSIONS; *spasms; eruptions; suppressed, from; scarlatina* (5)
GENERALS; CONVULSIONS; *spasms; extremities; perspiration, from suppressed foot sweat* (1)

One way to avoid suppression with our homeopathic treatment is by paying attention to the miasms. This allows us to consider a wider and deeper symptom picture so that we choose the correct remedy for the entire disease rather than just for the most prominent symptom.

Multiple Miasms

Many remedies have prominent psoric symptoms. *Calcarea carbonica* and *Sulphur* are two very clear ones. *Calcarea carbonica* is the most psoric remedy available, even more psoric than *Sulphur*. But even *Calcarea carbonica* is not 100 percent psoric. Look in James Tyler Kent's *Repertory of the Homeopathic Materia Medica* (*Kent's Repertory*) under "MIND; KILL, desire to." The sixth edition of *Kent's Repertory* lists 24 remedies. *Calcarea carbonica* is there in plain type. Poor, fearful, weak, sweating, cold, hungry *Calcarea* has a syphilitic tendency! It is primarily psoric with a little bit of syphilis in it. A *Calcarea carbonica* patient may tell you that she so deeply fears her mother-in-law that she would like to kill her. Go through *Kent's Repertory* and locate all of the rubrics that contain *Calcarea*, then look in the Materia Medica as well. Considering all the symptoms of *Calcarea carbonica*, you will find that it is roughly 96 percent psoric, perhaps 3 percent syphilitic, and the rest sycotic and tubercular.

Now look at *Sulphur* and consider its miasms—a lot of psora: redness, itching, difficulty standing, and burning—much more burning than in *Calcarea carbonica*. But *Sulphur* is also a remedy that goes to extremes. *Sulphur* boasts a lot, has a lot of heat, and is always studying everything. These extremes are sycotic. If we look deeper, we will find other behaviors in *Sulphur*. At a certain point, the patient may not eat or drink any more, may not bathe, may not comb his hair, and may sit in a little hut in the mountains, totally alone and always thinking. We would characterize this behavior of isolating himself as syphilitic.

In our modern population it would be a rare person who has only one miasm, and in our Materia Medica there is no remedy that addresses only one miasm.

We can apply this information to our patients. A patient may come to us who is fat, sweats, can't stand the cold, is a good worker on whom you can depend, loves eggs, is constipated, and trusts you very much. When asked about his fears, he says, "I'm very afraid of mice." We inquire further about his inner nature, and he says, "I almost don't dare tell you. Switch off the video. Don't write this down. Sometimes I get the idea that I have to kill my child. I'm sure I'll never do it, but I'm so unhappy about this idea." The homeopath says, "Thank you. Now we'll prescribe *Mercurius*." Is this correct? At the end of the consultation, the homeopath prescribes a syphilitic remedy because of a syphilitic symptom, even though the patient is psoric and *Calcarea carbonica* would have covered everything. But we can know this only if we study the remedies thoroughly in light of their miasmatic composition.

Every remedy has its own unique balance of two or more miasms. A few remedies, called tri-miasmatic, exhibit a fairly equal mix of symptoms from psora, syphilis, and sycosis. Tri-miasmatic remedies are often needed for patients whose symptoms manifest in this way—with characteristic symptoms equally balanced among these three miasms.

Symptoms as a Guide to the Miasms

To get curative results, we must discern the miasm picture that shows itself most strongly in our patient, choosing a remedy within that miasm picture that is most similar to the characteristic totality of the patient.

Let's look at this statement a little more thoroughly. All patients exhibit symptoms from more than one miasm, so how do we decide which miasm needs to be treated at any given time? This is a very good question and one that we will spend time discussing throughout our time together, as this is the basis of miasmatic prescribing and case management.

We have to start with the language of the vital force—symptoms. In homeopathy we are always looking for the **characteristic** symptoms that best represent the **totality** of the patient in his disease. Part of that totality is the miasm(s). We must clarify which miasm(s) is most strongly represented in our patient at any given time. Of course we are not strictly mathematical in our prescribing, but a mathematical analogy may help to illustrate this principle. Let's say that the patient's total number of characteristic symptoms in each miasm represents the weight of the miasm for this patient. Perhaps 80 percent of her symptoms are psoric, 15 percent are syphilitic, and 5 percent are sycotic. If so, then Psora is currently most prominent in her case, and we will do best to choose a remedy that has this same miasmatic distribution, namely a primarily psoric one.

To identify the miasm that any symptom represents, we must first understand each symptom in its entirety and in its context within the totality of the patient.

How do we determine which miasm is expressed in a given symptom? We must understand the nature and dynamics of each miasm, but we must also know how to assess the character of the symptom. Just as a particular diagnosis does not point to a particular remedy, a particular symptom does not necessarily point to a particular miasm. For example, asthma can be from any miasm. Psoric asthma has a psoric character, perhaps being brought on by exhaustion, cold weather, or fear. Sycotic asthma might be worse in damp; syphilitic asthma could be worse at night, with stabbing pains in the chest. The key to identifying the miasm of a particular symptom is in **how it is expressed** in the individual patient. Often it helps to study its etiology, modalities, and concomitants. In patients where two or more miasms are intertwined, a single symptom may exhibit characteristics of more than one miasm.

Most symptoms can be from any miasm, depending on their particular characteristics. Therefore when we study the miasms, we must learn the character, the dynamics of each miasm, not simply a list of symptoms.

Miasmatic Prescribing and Long-Term Case Management

Since all of our patients are multi-miasmatic, and since homeopathic treatment affects the miasms, the weight of the miasms will shift in our patients as they proceed toward cure. This shifting directs our subsequent prescriptions over time.

In the above example, for instance, our first remedy would be psoric and would calm the psoric miasm in her; later the syphilitic miasm, which we know is in her, might become more prominent, and then we might need to give a syphilitic remedy, when the time is right. Knowing from the beginning that syphilis is in her, we will not be tempted to give an "acute" remedy for the syphilitic symptoms, which would suppress them and cause the syphilitic miasm to become more deeply entrenched in her.

Sometimes when we as homeopaths find we are "chasing the symptoms," when our remedies each act "well" but we don't see a lasting improvement in the patient's overall health, it is because we have not understood the dynamics of the miasmatic picture. Each prescription may even shift the miasmatic picture somewhat, so that the patient looks different although not fundamentally improving. Many of our cases that we call "stalled," "confused," or "incurable" result from a history of this kind of treatment.

By paying attention to the miasmatic mix from the very beginning of a case, we can follow the case intelligently in the long term.

When homeopaths do not understand the miasmatic basis of disease, we give so many different remedies that there is little sense to our prescribing.

Patients may wind up with a long history of one remedy after another, and they are different, but not better than they were at the beginning. If we know the complete miasmatic picture, we will understand exactly why the case unfolds as it does over time.

All Homeopathic Treatment Addresses Miasms

It is a common misunderstanding that there is a difference between "treating the patient" (or using "the constitutional remedy") and "treating the miasm" (or using "a miasmatic remedy"). When we consider that the totality encompasses the miasmatic picture, how can we reasonably make this distinction? Another misunderstanding is that the nosodes address the miasms more directly than other remedies do. When we search through the Repertory and Materia Medica to identify the miasmatic composition of our remedies, we find that this too is inaccurate. *Calcarea carbonica,* for instance, has a higher percentage of psoric symptoms than *Psorinum.*

All treatment addresses miasms, and every remedy is a miasmatic remedy when it is accurately chosen with the miasms in view.

When prescribing with attention to the miasms, we are still looking for the simillimum—the remedy that best covers the totality of the case. The difference, when we add in the consideration of miasms, is that the totality is larger and our chance of finding the simillimum is greater. Let's look now at each of the five miasms individually, clarify how to recognize these miasmatic patterns in our patients, and learn how to apply our knowledge of the miasms to our cases so that we can treat our patients profoundly and well.

CHAPTER 1

Psora and the Psoric Miasm

All disease is due to one or more of the miasms. A large part of disease belongs to what Hahnemann called psora. He called it the "mother" of all diseases. No disease can exist without the foundation of psora. To fully cure a patient, we have to eventually treat psora.

What is psora? Originally, it was a kind of skin disease—an itch. It was quite innocent because one would have to scratch that itch but would never die from it. It caused suffering and restlessness. Whenever there is a history of itch, it belongs to psora. Hahnemann said it was an illness that could be seen on the skin. When the skin illness was suppressed, this activated the chronic internal disease or miasm of psora.

Mental and Emotional Symptoms and Expressions of the Psoric Miasm

Weakness
Too little
Not capable
Hard working
Care for others
Family oriented
Preparing
Saves things
Possessive
Wants to make a good impression
Slowness
Worry
Shyness
Blushing
Guilt
Desires safe, solid, long-lasting things
Softness
Quiet
Clinging
Dependent
Fearful
Ailments from fear
Impressionable

One prominent symptom of psora is **lack of energy**. "I always feel tired and have to rest" is a symptom of psora. The patient has the feeling that he is weak—mentally, emotionally, and physically. He may feel exhausted. He feels too weak to do things, but he has a lot of ideas about what he *will* do—next year when he is not so tired, has more money, or has a better diploma.

Psoric people have wonderful ideas about the future, but they do not do a lot today because they do not have the energy. Their minds are always active about tomorrow or next year. They may be daydreamers, building "castles in the air." The psoric homeopath says, "If only I had a few thousand dollars and a nice desk, then I could practice well." Psora has a lot of imagination. Some psoric patients work hard because of anxiety about their financial situation and security in the future, but this work exhausts them because of their psora.

Psora has the feeling of **having too little**—too little money, too little confidence, too little physical strength. When psora feels she does not have enough of something, what does she do? She wants more. She needs more to feel secure. How does she react mentally to the feeling of having too little? She compensates. Psora may say, "I have only one nice dress. I have to wash my dress and hang it outside, but I'd better watch it or somebody might take it." Psora's idea is "Whatever I have, someone might take it, and I will not be able to buy it again." When she has this feeling of poverty and believes that whenever she loses something she'll never be able to get it again, her reaction is to hold on tightly. She saves everything, and she worries. She is careful with her possessions and saves her money. She will not spend it now because next month she may need it.

Psora is attached to his **possessions**. He likes to collect things because of his feeling of not having enough (lack), and he may become greedy. Some patients complain about having only this or that, but sometimes, after they die, the newspaper reveals that they left behind a lot of money and possessions. These may be the same patients who felt they did not have enough money to pay for their homeopathic consultation.

If psora wants to travel, consider how she **prepares**. She takes a lot of money with her and puts everything in her suitcase, including warm clothes and snacks. She is the best person to travel with. She does not need to buy a lot on the trip because she has planned so thoroughly and brought along every possible thing she might need. If she does buy something, it is something that she considers seriously beforehand. In Belgium we say, "She turns around every penny."

Calcarea carbonica is a primarily psoric remedy, so let's discuss her psoric expressions. *Calcarea carbonica* fears she might not be able to continue working long enough to take care of herself, so she **saves** just in case. *Calcarea* *carbonica* needs support and strength, and she eats to get it—high-calorie foods such as eggs, meat, cheese, and pastry. She needs energy to become strong enough to work and earn money for the future.

Calcarea carbonica **works and works** and works. She may work until she is 73 years old and has no more strength, and even then she will want to be doing something, so strong is the need to be sure she has enough. There is a nice rubric: **MIND; AVERSION;** ***everything, to; sits idle, as soon as he.*** *Calcarea* is the only remedy. *Nux vomica* is also a psoric remedy, but *Nux vomica* earns money because he likes the feeling of power that money gives him, while *Calcarea carbonica* works and earns money so that she can save enough for herself and for others. *Calcarea carbonica* avoids a lot of spending and calculates how she can get the most for her money. *Nux vomica* does not spend much money on others, but for himself he likes the best wine and the best restaurants—for his wife and children, not so much. *Nux vomica* wants to retire in the future, therefore he works but not steadily. He works efficiently in bursts and then rests. Both are weak, and both are affected by too much work. Although *Calcarea carbonica* works like an elephant and *Nux vomica* like a cheetah, both are psoric remedies, needing the comfort of money.

Psora is the mother of all **anxieties and fears**—fear of death, fear that something will happen, fear about finances, and so on. Although most of the psoric patient's physical complaints are worse during the day, he tends to notice his anxiety more at night. During the day he is busy and distracted, but at night when his mind stops to rest, he worries and is anxious. When he is totally alone and in the dark, he begins to reflect, recall the day, and worry, and then the fears come out. Psoric children do not think about their fears in the daylight, but as soon as the darkness comes, all the dogs and dragons come to mind. Often, **fears come on at night** before they fall asleep. Psora may be afraid of the dark, robbers, strangers, big dogs, illness, accidents, and death; of something happening to his loved ones, speaking in public, and being alone; and of the future and other unknown situations. Psora has many fears. Having **ailments from fear** is psoric. A psoric patient may be too shy or too embarrassed to admit his fears readily—he has so many—but ask him to tell you a story about something that touched him—his biggest fear or grief—and these fears come out.

If psora thinks about stealing something, it will be to fill some need. But then he worries, "If I steal, they might put me in jail." His mind is extremely active. He considers the results of his actions. He thinks about everything. In Belgium the expression is, "He counts every step he makes." When psora tells a lie, it is because of his fear of being punished, humiliated, or embarrassed. He is sensitive to reprimand and feels shame and guilt easily.

How does psora sleep? He feels tired in the morning, because during the night he is thinking about his problems, about everything he has to do tomorrow. He **worries**, "How is my bank account?" "What will I say to my mother?" "Should I do this thing or that thing?" **Irresolution** is psoric. The thinking is boring and tiring, but he cannot stop. His mind is going all night. How will he get through the next day? Psora would like to have 10 hours of sleep, and sometimes even that is not enough. Psora may dream of being paralyzed or of **not being able** to find something or do something in his dreams. The psoric homeopath may dream of being unable to find the correct remedy for his patient. His patient is dying because he cannot find the remedy. Perhaps he fears that he will give the wrong remedy and hurt his patient in some way. Psora is anxious and dreams about her fear. Her nightmares are about all the things she worries about during the day—thoughts of failed efforts, frustration, and incapacity. This is the psoric night.

We should always ask our patients what kind of **dreams** they have. This helps us understand what the uncompensated mind is dealing with during the night. The feelings one struggles to control in the day come out at night. Dreams can help the vital force overcome problems. They may disturb one's sleep, but dreams help get things out. The correct remedy will speed up this process of getting things out.

Psora cannot stand violence. Psora does not watch violent films or read violent stories because the images haunt her. She gets anxious. She has to turn off a scary movie or news program or hide her eyes. She cannot get rid of the awful images of things she has heard and seen. The rubric **MIND; HORRIBLE things;** ***sad stories affect her profoundly*** is a psoric rubric. Because of her **impressionability** and her imagination, psora is deeply affected by witnessing frightening events. There is an antidepressant currently on the market with the potential side effect of violent action toward oneself or others. Some patients have actually killed themselves while on this drug. This would never be a psoric reaction.

Psora likes happy endings. She likes love stories and romantic notions. She may have feelings of being unloved, forsaken, sad, or lonely. She fears being alone. Psora likes **consolation** and will ask for **support**. She needs company and may become dependent on others. Psora may even behave childishly. In some marriages, a psoric woman may be treated badly by her husband or partner, even beaten, and yet she may not leave him. She feels that she **cannot defend herself**. She may be afraid that he will find her and beat her up even more or that she will never be able to make it on her own. This is a psoric reaction. A sycotic wife would give her husband a beating in return.

Psora has trouble making decisions. If he decides one thing, he has to let another thing go, and he does not like to let go. Psora holds on to his possessions. He does not like things that change. He buys **classic** clothing. Psora may keep a once fashionable shawl for 40 years. It may have gone out of fashion long ago, but she thinks that the style may come back, so she holds on to it.

How do psoric people behave sexually? They say, "I am too tired," or they are shy about it. **Shyness** is psoric. Coition may cause itch and other problems afterward for women. They may scratch until it burns. Males may not be able to have an erection because of weakness. Females may have infertility due to weakness. During the sexual act, psoric patients may complain of being cold. A girl may feel pressured to have sex in her early teenage years just because she wants to please her partner and not lose him. She may think, "All the girls in school have already had sex, and I am the only one who hasn't." She fears being judged by others. She wants to be accepted. What is her psoric reaction to abuse or rape? She feels shame. Her body may stop developing because of fear. She may think, "I cannot have another sexual relationship, and I cannot tell anyone." When psora is jealous, it will be from worry of losing her partner because she depends on him.

When we see a patient in the waiting room, we can get a first impression of his miasm. Psora looks shy, timid, bashful, and afraid to make contact. His face may be **flushed**. When someone speaks to him, he is happy. Psora wants to talk, but he is mostly timid. When we speak with a psoric patient, how does he express himself? He says things such as, "I'm sorry. Did I disturb you?" He likes to give his answers precisely. He wants to give correct answers. He tries to make a **good impression**. He wants people to think good things about him. This is a psoric concern.

When we observe a psoric patient, what do we see? We may see either paleness or redness in the skin; the psoric miasm has both. Her lips may be very red as in the remedy *Sulphur*. Psora dresses to be warm. She likes to be covered up. Psora tends to wear neat, plain, unassuming clothing—often light blue, gray, or beige. She **does not want to stand out**. How does psora sit? He slouches, leans on the table, or slides down in his chair. *Sulphur* is a psoric remedy that cannot sit up straight; he **slumps** because he does not have the strength to straighten his body. He has to lean on something, and he cannot stand for long periods.

When psora has to speak in front of others, he is very timid, too shy to say anything. Sometimes we see overcompensation in psoric patients. We often see someone who is acting too extroverted, telling everybody everything. A psoric person may use alcohol to compensate so that he can overcome his shyness and be able to talk. But if he is very psoric and drinks too much, he may fall asleep.

It is not what happens in somebody's life, but how he or she reacts to it, that is important in determining the homeopathic prescription.

We must try to be objective, keep our own reactions out of the consultation, and watch what is going on with the patient so that we can treat the symptoms of the patient and not our own symptoms or our own reactions. All people feel fear, anger, and sadness. What people do with these feelings—how they react, how they compensate, how they express their feelings—are the characteristics that point to the miasm. How someone reacts to life's events provides the homeopath with that person's characteristic symptoms. A psoric patient may **feel paralyzed** by fear and be unable to fight the fear. He may feel that he is a coward. When a psoric patient is angry, he simmers, feels guilty, and gets a red face but does not do anything. He feels blocked and is speechless. If an injustice is done to him, he suffers it inside. How is **psoric grief**? There is moaning, weeping, and talking with someone who will listen. This is a normal grief. But psora does not talk to just anybody; he talks to the people with whom he feels safe, people who will understand and will not judge him.

Most **guilt** is psoric. Psora talks about her guilt only with people who are close to her. She is sympathetic, and sometimes she does not feel appreciated enough. She may be conscientious about trifles and painstaking in her behavior. A psoric homeopath will work very hard. She may worry about her prescription all night: "Do I have the right remedy? Have I thought of everything?" She may be very dogmatic, sticking to one philosophy, not being able to work with "open eyes." Psora may be fastidious, because a neighbor might see that her windows are not clean enough. She needs the good opinion of others. She gets anxious about trifles. Timidity, lack of confidence, embarrassment, bashfulness, nervousness, and worry are psoric. Psora may bite her nails down to the point where they are very painful, all because of worry.

Everything you see in a patient tells about his state and, ultimately, his miasm. Observe. Do not be prejudiced. Challenge yourself. Understand your patient.

A patient's profession can tell a lot about him. What professions does psora fancy? Perhaps nursing. We might suppose that policemen would not be psoric, but I have treated some. One officer I treated was very fearful. Every time he had to write a ticket, he began to tremble and was afraid someone would notice his trembling. **Trembling** is a psoric reaction. Sometimes people choose professions that are contrary to their basic feelings to overcome these feelings and fears. Always ask why about a behavior. Everything tells the state of a patient. What kind of art does he like? What kind of books does he read? How does he dress? We must try to recognize the state in every situation. Psoric people usually like steady, stable jobs from which they can retire after many years of working for the same employer. They may like jobs with lots of **rules and fixed positions**, such as bureaucratic jobs. If they are joggers, they are running because of concern for their health.

The patient's miasm is expressed in every aspect of his life, and we can confirm the miasm in all actions, reactions, and even the personal choices he makes.

Consider psora when he is buying a car. He will go to every shop and look at every car, study the insurance costs, and see which car gets the best mileage and uses the least oil. Finally, he will buy a **safe**, **solid**, **long-lasting** car. Not necessarily the cheapest, but a classic, because he can sell it for more money later. He considers its investment value. The color may be a quiet, **soft** gray or blue. Psora's dog of choice will be a strong one for protection or a cuddly one for company.

Psoric patients **complain** of various physical ailments, but they live into their 80s or 90s. The life expectancy of psoric patients is long. In Belgium we say, "Long-lasting cars always creak." Psoric patients may talk about their complaints, but they live a long time. They have many anxieties about their health. They fear that a lump may be cancer. They get the flu and fear they may die from it. They suffer from headaches, sleeping problems, poor digestion, stomach pains, and restlessness. They may go to the doctor, get a blood test, and find out they lack iron. But the psoric problem will not be a cancer that metastasizes quickly or a bleeding ulcer. **Psoric problems are functional**. The psoric miasm generally does not cause serious disturbances in the tissues, but these patients are anxious about their health anyway. They may despair of recovering. Psora wants the homeopath's support, and she may spend hours in consultation. She likes having a homeopath listen to her. She likes to consult medical books and study the body. She checks the Internet and comes to the homeopath with a list of remedies to ask which one suits her. There is also a lot of psora in homeopaths and in other health care workers.

Psora needs to **feel safe**. While sycosis likes the city for the activity and the nightlife and syphilis likes to live apart from other people, psora likes a quiet neighborhood for protection, with a grocery store nearby. Psora also buys insurance against every disaster.

Psora **does not assimilate well**—nutrients, the personalities of other people, or certain ideas. There is a weakness about absorbing natural things and a weakness about throwing off harmful things. It is a weakness in reaction. The weakness affects psora at the mental, emotional, and physical levels. Psora's memory may be weak, and he may be forgetful. Psora's mind is usually quick and active, but he may also be slow to learn due to weakness.

General and Physical Symptoms and Modalities of the Psoric Miasm

Weakness
Functional disturbances
Clear or white, bland discharges
Daytime problems

Assimilation issues
Dentition problems
Eruptions
Itching, burning, dryness
Softness, smoothness, roundness, pinkness
Pedunculated growths
Mollusca
Sourness
Coldness
Movement aggravates
Rest ameliorates
Eating
Building (structure, security)
Drowsiness
Conservation
Desires sweets and warmth

Psora **itches**. The itching of psora is remarkable, and he is forever scratching to relieve the itch. But the more psora **scratches**, the more he itches. Then the itch starts to **burn**, and then it hurts. It may be a strong itch. He lies in bed and itches and scratches until he feels mad. While he is worrying about money, family, his house, and what he has to do tomorrow, he is scratching.

Psora has many **skin** problems. Few nutrients get to the skin, and the skin is dry. The **dryness** and itching are worse in the daytime, from the heat of the bed, and from bathing. **Eruptions** that itch or burn are usually psoric. Acne is psoric when boils come up with no discharges and go away slowly. Psora's ears may be dry, itchy, and scaly. Psoric crusts and scabs are **light and fine**. We think of warts as sycotic, but they may also be psoric; it depends on how they manifest. Psoric warts are soft and smooth and only a little bit elevated. They are round and fleshy, mostly skin-colored or a little pink, and soft to the touch. They also may be flat and dry and may itch. Mollusca presenting as soft balls, flesh-colored, close together, and usually in clusters, are psoric. Psoric mollusca are soft, weak, and not active and have been there for a long time. Most of the mollusca I see in my practice resolve nicely with *Calcarea carbonica*. Pedunculated warts (warts with little stems) are psoric. A psoric ulcer is bright red with burning pain. The psoric ulcer ripens slowly and heals slowly.

Psora feels her physical problems most strongly in the **daytime** and feels **worse when the sun is highest in the sky**. Psoric aggravation climbs according to the intensity of the sun. Psora may have a fever in the morning that is worse at noon. Her energy begins to drop, and she usually feels tired in the middle of the day. The heat of the sun makes psora suffer, but she cannot stand the cold either. She cannot tolerate a **draft** or air conditioning. She has an aversion to cold **wind**, but even warm wind gives her a sensation she does not like. Psora is worse from drafts, wind, and cold. There is a **basic weakness** of the nervous system and **oversensitivity** to sounds, sights, and smells. Psora may be very irritable because of this oversensitivity.

Psoric patients are **cold**. They have cold hands and feet. When the psoric homeopath sits on his comfortable couch with his central heating and reads *Kent's Repertory*, his feet and hands get cold. He has to turn up the heat, but he still does not feel warm. A feeling of cold water running on the leg or on the body is psoric. This feeling is due to deficiency. Psora is generally **better from warmth**.

Psora sweats. Any miasm can have sweating, but psora **sweats from weakness** and from an **inability to adapt quickly** or to distribute his internal heat properly. There is sweating in the night. It is normal for someone to sweat during exercise, but sweating when at rest—in bed, for example—is psoric. One clue to recognizing psora in the consulting room is to observe its **unique smell**, if the natural odor has not been covered by deodorant or perfume. However, in the sophisticated world of today, there are few natural smells but many artificial ones. Companies sell strong-smelling products to cover or eliminate natural body odors. TV commercials promote hundreds of products that we can buy to cover up our human "weaknesses." We repair our teeth, straighten our bites, buy artificial nails, color our hair, smooth our wrinkles, and wash away our bad breath and body odor. But homeopaths sometimes have the privilege of being in a consulting room for an hour or more with a sick, smelly patient. The psoric patient has a **sour smell**. Not only is the perspiration sour, but also the breath smells sour. Other discharges, including the stool, smell sour as well. Psora feels better from discharges such as perspiration, urination, and diarrhea. Psoric discharges are **thin and watery, clear or white, and bland** or a little bit sour. Psoric asthma has **mucus like clear water**.

Psora comes to the homeopath with a history of being weak and tired. She cannot climb mountains. She can't even climb stairs easily. Some people ascend stairs by skipping steps, but psora clings to the handrail all the way, breathing with difficulty. Psora may get tired after half a dance. **Exertion aggravates** her problems. She can't do a lot of exercise because she starts to sweat more. It is not only the physical body that has difficulty but also the emotional and mental areas. Psora feels that she will never have the strength to do certain things. She says, "If I had your energy, I'd be able to do this or that."

One way we can get more energy when we feel we don't have enough is to eat! The psoric patient fills up to get more strength. He needs his food. He **cannot wait to eat**. He may nibble in the morning. He wants lots of rich, heavy food for energy—meat, milk, eggs, and fatty foods. He eats to try to overcome his feeling of weakness, and he may become obese because of this. Psora likes sweets and warm foods. He eats large quantities and may be very thirsty. Psora may have the unusual desire to eat indigestible things—chalk, fingernails, clinkers (boogers), and scabs. Sometimes psora may describe a burnt taste in his mouth.

When psora eats, she may have problems due to weak digestion. Her **digestion is slow**. There is often a history of constipation and symptoms of poor nutrition. Once a psoric patient has taken a psoric remedy, she can assimilate nutrients better. The remedy stimulates her vital force so she can digest food and assimilate essential nutrients. Healthy bodies are wonderful! For people who live at the North Pole and eat mostly fish or who live in Asia and eat mostly rice, their healthy bodies can manufacture what they need to function well with the foods that nature supplies.

Psora experiences many **disturbances of sensation and function**. Fainting and vertigo belong to psora. He has sensations of dizziness. His eyes are sensitive to light. There may be spots before his eyes. His eyesight tends to become weaker and weaker. He is sensitive to smells. He may have sensations of tingling or numbness in the skin. Most of the **"as if" sensations** in *Kent's Repertory* belong to psora.

Psora has very dry, thin hair that breaks easily. His hair may have a strange appearance—it **tangles**; the Repertory uses the word "matted." He may have a dry, itchy scalp. His hair may be white in spots.

Psora may have poor nails and teeth because of insufficient absorption of minerals from her diet. Her nails are weak and bend or break easily. Her teeth are soft, may be smaller than they should be, and get smaller as the surface wears away. **Psoric teeth** require fillings on the top surfaces. The dentist tells psora that she must be grinding her teeth, because the enamel is being worn away. Psora may have osteoporosis and brittle bones that break. She is unable to absorb enough calcium for her bones to be strong.

Hypofunctions such as low blood pressure and slow pulse and heartbeat are psoric when they are due to a weakness. The psoric patient has sensations and worries about his heart without having heart disease. Although he worries about his health, the psoric miasm alone does not cause serious disturbances in the tissues.

In general, the psoric state produces illnesses that are characterized by a situation or feeling of **weakness** or **too little**. There isn't enough energy to produce a strong picture of disease.

Every symptom and every illness must be looked at in context.

How does the body respond to illness? What are the modalities? With that in mind, the following discussion addresses some of the psoric illnesses I see in my consulting room.

A psoric lung inflammation **comes on slowly**, with a low-grade fever. Patients with these lung inflammations cough and do not feel well, and the cough does not go away. The lung infection may not be easy to detect because the symptoms are not strong. Often, the infection can be discovered only by taking an x-ray. Psora is often too weak to have clear symptoms. After vaccinations, psora may have a chronic fatigue reaction, because psora's innate weakness cannot withstand the insult of vaccination.

A psoric ear infection also **comes on slowly** and with little fever. The discharge is bland and watery. A psoric ear infection never destroys the ear or causes deafness.

With psoric flu, there is chilliness, low energy, and a need for more sleep that may go on for some days before the illness breaks out. The fever is dragging and low, not high.

If a psoric person gets a stomach ulcer, it may take years of burning, burping, and heaviness in the stomach for the ulcer to develop. Sometimes there is discomfort, sometimes not. When the doctor finally sends him to the hospital and an ulcer is found, the psoric patient may fear he has cancer. He worries about why the ulcer developed. In psora, it may be due to his **constant worrying**—about his future or whether he is performing well enough in his job. His boss tells him he is too slow, but really it is psora's need to do it correctly, carefully, so that he makes a good impression, that he takes his time. Psora feels that he *might not be capable,* so he works extra hard to show that he *is capable.* It is not slowness as in dullness—it is that psora is careful to be seen as doing things well. This is the quality that shoots to his need for a psoric remedy.

With psoric appendicitis, there is pain, but also doubt on the part of the doctor as to its etiology. If the patient's psoric weakness is such that he does not have enough energy to produce strong and clear symptoms of an acute appendix, the pain may last for days or months. Without a clear picture, the doctor may be unsure how to diagnose and treat him.

Psora has muscle aches and pains and various kinds of neuralgia. These pains are **worse from cold and movement** and **worse during the day**. He feels better from rest and warmth. Pain caused by too much movement is psoric. Psora feels weakness after exertion. His muscles lack tone, and he may have awkwardness. Standing is very hard for psora. He will not be able to stand for long periods without becoming restless because of his weakness.

Involuntary urination is psoric because of the weakness of the muscles, although urinary problems in general are sycotic. Psora may have problems with either diarrhea or constipation. Intestinal worms also are psoric.

The Psoric Miasm in Infants and Children

Psoric babies may be **drowsy** at birth. They are **timid**, **fearful**, **clinging**, and **dependent** on the mother and **want to be held**, with fear of falling. They are always hungry and crying and have skin eruptions with itching and scratching. When someone holds a little baby, she usually has a nice smell. Psoric babies **smell sour**; even their feet are stinky. These are the babies for whom companies make baby powder. A baby should be warm, but psoric babies are **cold** and cannot be warmed up. This is a strange, rare, and peculiar symptom for a baby. The common illnesses of psoric babies are snuffles, colds, cradle cap, and ear infections, with a little moistness behind the eardrum. As children, they are weak and somewhat smaller than average. They may have growth problems or may remain smaller than normal. Dentition may be **late and slow**, and they may walk later than expected.

An ear infection in psoric children has a slow onset and a weak response, with some pain and fever; the ear is **a little red** inside. The child does not feel well. He complains and is irritable, with a desire to be with his mother. He cries and weeps several times a day about his earache. He plays and then comes back for a little bit of comfort. Mostly, the ear is not burning. A psoric child with an ear infection needs warmth or puts his hand on his ear.

Dentition is often difficult for psoric babies and children. They may have **difficulty in forming teeth** because of weakness. They may be **late** in getting new teeth, and the baby teeth are **slow** to fall out. Their teeth may decay due to lack of silica absorption. If these **weak children** are given allopathic silica and strong indigestible minerals, the stool becomes white and the children become constipated because their bodies **cannot assimilate** the minerals. Correct homeopathic care will address the weakness of psora—the inability to absorb or assimilate will improve, and then the condition of the teeth can improve. Otherwise, all the added minerals will only go into the toilet.

Imagine Baby Psora's early life. He is very dependent, cold, with cold feet, and has a kind of weakness; he is **easily disturbed** and **easily tired**, with a weakness in digesting his mother's milk. He has been treated with antibiotics, and he gets indigestion and (hopefully) diarrhea, because a discharge is good. But another allopathic prescription will stop the diarrhea. The child has the tendency to be weak, so now he develops asthma or breathing difficulties.

Another scenario for Baby Psora might be **snuffles**, which, when treated with antibiotics, results in subsequent weakness, followed by more snuffles and repeated antibiotics, resulting in more weakness. Then he starts to get throat infections. These too are treated with antibiotics, but now there are no snuffles anymore. Instead, moisture appears in the eustachian tube, and repeated ear infections develop, which are treated with more antibiotics. Because the doctor is unable to cure or prevent these infections, she may decide to operate and put tubes in the baby's ears. The baby develops repeated tonsillitis, and then his tonsils are removed. What is the result? The best response Baby Psora can produce is laryngitis or croup. What does the doctor do then? She gives more drugs. The child becomes weaker and weaker because of psora, but his psoric miasm never gets treated.

Now imagine that the same Baby Psora is born and his mother says, "I will not suffer with my child." She goes to a homeopath for the snuffles. The homeopath asks questions about the pregnancy and the baby. Is the baby hot or cold? How is his stool? Does he perspire on his head? Does he have cold feet? Does he drink a lot? Does he like to lie down on his abdomen? Is there a sour smell of stool? The homeopath hears "yes" to these questions. What is the prescription? *Calcarea carbonica.* What happens? The child gets stronger—although the snuffles may go on for a while—but the child continues to grow stronger and gets over the snuffles with no problems.

I have much experience in treating babies, and to my astonishment, almost every baby from age six weeks to three months has skin eruptions. Why? They are clearing out the psora.

This is the body's way of bringing the miasm to the surface and getting rid of it. Without knowing that this is the best possible "healing process" a baby can produce, parents and doctors often apply creams that suppress these eruptions, which causes psora to be driven back inside, and the struggle continues. In many countries when babies are three months old, if not earlier, they are vaccinated, further weakening their ability to discharge psora.

Children's diseases are now coming out in the form of eczema, which is much more difficult to cure than simple eruptions.

What's going on? The struggle goes deeper and deeper. We are on the way to having very ill children. When children in my practice have a childhood disease and they are on a constitutional remedy, it helps them and they have no complications from the illness. I do not touch the illness with another homeopathic remedy. I let it come out naturally. They are not that ill. The reaction is quick and strong in coming out, and they do not suffer that much; it is the parents who suffer. The same is true with itching or eruptions in little children. The parents suffer more than the child does, especially when well-meaning friends, family members, or teachers tell them, "You should take that child to the pediatrician or dermatologist."

Psoric children go to the parents' bed to sleep because of **fear**. They are **timid** and **shy** when they have to recite at school. They are sensitive and are hurt if scolded or reprimanded by their teachers. They **need support** from the family. When they see something frightening on television, they cover their eyes and have nightmares. As with psoric adults, psoric children may be very keen of mind (which is often the case), slow to learn, or deficient in mental ability. When seen in a psoric child, this slowness or deficiency is due to the weakness of psora rather than to the destruction of ability resulting from a syphilitic influence.

Children show what they are thinking and feeling through their play. Ask the parents to tell you how their children play. Psoric children are able to play quietly with concentration and focus.

Psoric Remedies

When studying the remedies, how do we know whether a remedy is a psoric remedy? In the modern repertories in the Generals section, there is the rubric "Psora." In *Kent's Repertory*, under "GENERALITIES," there are "Syphilis" and "Sycosis" rubrics but nothing for psora. Only three miasms were considered at the time *Kent's Repertory* was written, and the remedies not listed under "Syphilis" or "Sycosis" were predominantly psoric. A good way to learn remedies by their miasms is to analyze what percentages of the remedy's symptoms are psoric, syphilitic, or sycotic.

> *We need only know the symptoms of the miasms to be able to classify the symptoms of the remedies. In simple terms, we can begin to classify most symptoms by what is too little (psoric), too much (sycotic), or destructive (syphilitic).*

A nosode is a potentized remedy prepared from diseased tissue. *Psorinum*, prepared from the scabies vesicle, is the nosode of the psoric miasm. Here are some of the psoric symptoms in *Psorinum*:

- Tremendous anxiety
- Fear of poverty
- Lack of energy
- Forsaken feeling
- Chilly
- Aggravated from cold
- Ailments from suppressed eruptions
- Sensitive to drafts
- Constant hunger, better eating

- Itching
- Skin eruptions

Psora Case 1: Boy With Cough and Delayed Growth

Video Presentation and Case Description

The following discussion was captured as it occurred during a video presentation and case description by Henny Heudens. Student questions and comments appear in brackets. In the interview portions, "HH" indicates a question or comment by Henny, and "P" indicates the patient's comment or response.

This slender boy with brown hair is answering very timidly and sweetly. He looks to his mother sometimes before answering. If you know my voice well, you see how softly I am speaking in this interview. He is 12 years old, and later you will see how small, sweet, and weak he is. He looks more like six or seven years old. In the consultation, I am asking him about his sleep. He answers very correctly. What do you see? [*He does not have much eye contact.*] [*He is apprehensive.*] [*His chin is tucked down as if shying away from you.*] He is very timid and slow moving. His voice is very soft. You feel like you want to put your arm around him and say, "You are a sweet boy."

I saw this boy because he is always coughing, has had croup several times, and is backward (delayed) in growth. He has also suffered earaches, skin problems, and wetting his pants. He is without enough strength to cope with school life. He hates school. He has a sister one-and-a-half years younger. What is going on with him? When his sister was a toddler, there was no problem, but she is growing up now and is the big boss of her older brother, both physically and emotionally. She tells him what to do. Those of you who are small in size know what happens in this situation. You might become shy and withdrawn, perhaps mostly a reader all your life. Maybe you become an extrovert, but inside you still feel shyness. When you do something publicly and feel shy inside, the next night or day you might think, "What did I say?" or "What did I do in front of others." All of us have a *little* of this.

Where is his weakness? Everywhere—physically and emotionally. Imagine him in a class with strong boys. He hates school, not because he doesn't want to learn but because he cannot cope with the stronger boys. His skin is very pale, and he is very sweet and delicate.

He has been treated with:

- *Causticum* (cough a little better)
- *Phosphorus* (cough a little better)
- *Pulsatilla* (amelioration for a short time and then nothing)
- *Silica* (nothing)
- *Mercury* (nothing)
- *Tuberculinum* (amelioration then nothing)
- *Syphilinum*
- *Ferrum phosphoricum* (helped earache)
- *Sulphur*
- *Tuberculinum aviara*
- *Baryta carbonica* 30C (a little better), then 200C (worked one day and worse again)
- *Natrum muriaticum* (stopped wetting pants but no reaction on earache or retarded growth)
- *Staphysagria* (nothing)
- *Graphites* (skin a little better but cough unchanged)
- *Spongia* (cough a little better)

It is interesting that this psoric boy had never been given *Psorinum.* His is a classic case of psora with no long-lasting reaction to any other remedy. He did not get *Psorinum* at this moment either, and if he had there would have been no result. I will explain later.

He has had croup since he was three years old. We remember that his sister is one-and-a-half years younger. Did his problems have something to do with the birth of his sister? When a child is so small in size, it is important to know why. What happened? During the pregnancy, there was conflict in the family, and the mother endured much crying and sadness. During the pregnancy and the birth, she felt very helpless. During the birth, she felt that she could not make decisions for herself but that other people always decided for her—thus, the helpless feeling. During birth, she had very high blood pressure, and the doctors were trying to get the baby out as quickly as possible. After birth, the baby cried a lot. There was a lot of pain in his abdomen, and he was very dissatisfied and liked to be fed every 30 minutes. He was very hungry. He swallowed the milk quickly, with much appetite.

He was vaccinated against tuberculosis (TB) when he was three days old, had a tetanus vaccination at eight months of age, and when he was three years old he started to wet his pants (until he was 10 years old). We hear now why he was given *Tuberculinum.* His mother thought he started to cough because of the TB vaccination. He was given:

- *Causticum* (enuresis)
- *Natrum muriaticum* (abandoned feeling of the mother)
- *Pulsatilla* (crying of the mother)
- *Syphilinum*

I asked about the family background. The family background shows heart problems and hypertension, osteoporosis, stiffness of the joints, severe varicose veins, cancer, schizophrenia, and suicide, together with tuberculosis.

The first words his mother says are, "He is so helpless. He cannot do anything, and he does not take any initiative. He is the smallest in his class, and he lets every boy or girl in his class have power over him. He is so weak that when his sister watches movies on TV, he runs away crying. He cannot see things even made for children because he is so sensitive." His mother adds, "He is a nice child, and we love each other very much. When I feel sad and have tears in my eyes or I am crying, he comes to me and comforts me. He says, 'Mom, be happy.' He does not like it when I am weak."

The boy likes gymnastics, reads religious books, and likes to hear stories about heroes of the past. He likes to read thick books, the thicker the better. He likes to read about Indians. He likes to build houses in the woods outside. He likes to play alone. Now we think of *Natrum muriaticum,* and we think that maybe he was given the wrong potency.

He cannot sleep; it takes a long time before he falls asleep.

HH—Why?

P—Because I start to sweat, and I don't like sweating. Then I push away the covers, and I feel cold. I have the choice to sweat or suffer from the cold. This is why I can't sleep.

HH—Is this the only reason why you cannot sleep?

P—No, I am always thinking in my bed about what has happened or what I have seen or read. Once I fall asleep, I awake very easily.

His mother says that when she goes to the toilet at night, she is especially quiet because the smallest noise wakes him. When he was wetting the bed, his mother tried to wake him during the night to go to the toilet, and she says, "He was so friendly I could wake him up, and he'd always be so lovely and sweet." Too nice for the outside world!

How about his appetite? He likes soup, salmon (but not other fish), grapes, fruit, and cold drinks (without ice). He has nausea and does not like foods that contain milk. He drinks tea in the morning. He has an allergy to wasp stings (gets big swellings). He fears children who are bigger than he is. When he plays, he plays with small children.

He has a fear of watching television; he covers his eyes with his hands and weeps about little things. When he goes to school, he asks his mother what he'll eat at noon. If she tells him one thing, and then changes her mind, he starts to weep because she had promised to make something else. He has one idea, and when she changes it, he is disappointed.

HH—What would you like to be when you grow up? (His parents are in the medical profession.)

P—I'd like to be a server in a restaurant.

HH—Why?

P—I like people.

His mother says he likes food, likes to cook, and is very interested in food. Unlike his sister, he comes into the kitchen, looking into the pots, asking his mother what she added to make it so good.

HH—Does he only play outside and build houses?

Mother—No, he likes to play with little houses, little animals, and other tiny things. When I go shopping with him and his sister, she will choose something big, but he finds the tiniest things.

I ask how he behaves with animals, and she says he plays with little mice. He always likes to be very early when he goes someplace. He fears being late, and he is always pushing his mother to go. He does not like to be late, and this is the only problem between him and his mother. He has herpes on his lips, and this is because he is always biting his lips. He does this when something bores him. He likes hot food; likes to move, climb, and swing; and always likes to wear a hat. This is the whole case. We have to find the remedy that works for him.

Psora Case 1—Analysis

Before we solve the case, we must find out what is strange, rare, and peculiar. What is strange in this case? [*Desire to play with tiny little things.*] Yes; this is the idea that runs through the whole case—**smallness**, **childishness**, and **feeling small**. He is small physically and emotionally. Is he backward? No, he is not foolish; he is clever. How do we know? He reads very thick books, and he is interested in the past (heroes, Indians). Why? Because they are strong. He likes to read about strength because he is small. What is another interest? Cooking. It is strange for a young boy to be so interested in food. He likes special food. There is rigidity in him; he gets fixed ideas. It is difficult for him to change or go along with new ideas. He is not flexible but has his own way of doing things. There is stubbornness in him.

What about the profession he desires? Fireman and policeman are professions often chosen to compensate for weakness and show strength. This boy likes food, but he also likes to please. How better to please people than by serving them? A waiter can come close to people, see how they eat, and hear what they're talking about without the need to mix. One can be invisible in a certain way. What about his reading? This is somewhat abnormal for someone 12 years old. Most children do not spend so much time reading thick books because of their interest in television, except when TV is restricted.

What was one of his interests? Religion. When do most people become interested in religion? Six or seven years old, as in his case, would seem very young to be so interested in religion. Most people get interested in religion when they become independent from their parents, when they start to ask questions about life. Philosophical children ask questions (*Sulphur*, for example), but this boy is not like that. He does not ask a lot of questions, but he thinks a lot.

He likes gymnastics. Why? Because gymnastics involves motion and increases one's strength. So we know this case is an example of psora. Where do you see the weakness of psora? Everywhere. We see coldness. Also, he sweats at night. We see the smallness and shyness everywhere. If he were bigger, he would not have such a problem with going to school.

Now we go to the remedy. It has to be one with all of his strange, rare, and peculiar symptoms. These are:

- Likes tiny things
- Likes mice
- Interested in food
- Interested in religious books
- Rigidity, stubbornness
- Disappointments
- Fearful, weepy about scary things
- Cowers from powerful things

Rubrics

- MIND; HORRIBLE things; *sad stories affect her profoundly*
- MIND; RELIGIOUS; *affections, general; children, in*
- MIND; ANXIETY; *trifles, about*
- MIND; WEEPING, tearful mood; general; *easily*
- MIND; FEAR; general; *happen; something will*
- SLEEP; SLEEPLESSNESS; general; *thoughts, from*
- SLEEP; SLEEPLESSNESS; general; *noise, from slight*
- GENERALITIES; DWARFISHNESS

When you consider these rubrics, you come to one remedy, *Calcarea carbonica,* the most psoric remedy we have, even more psoric than *Psorinum,* which was asked about earlier and which does not cover the symptoms as well as *Calcarea* does.

Why did he get a lot of other remedies but not *Calcarea carbonica*? Because he was thin, with dark hair. If he had been obese and pale, with blue eyes, everyone would have prescribed *Calcarea.* Sometimes we mistakenly limit our remedy prescriptions by how our patients look on the outside, rather than relying on the totality of their disturbance. I gave him *Calcarea* 200C because this is a potency that matched his energy.

When patients are very, very weak, I prescribe lower; when very strong, I prescribe higher. I found it strange that he did not get this remedy, but I think the only reason was because he was small and dark, not obese and fair.

[*Why did you use "Horrible things, sad stories affect profoundly" if the things that bothered him so much were not so horrible? This rubric makes me think that an awful bloody accident would affect him. Why should watching the movie Bambi, for example, affect him?*]

Another patient told me of seeing *Bambi* when he was four years old. He told of remembering the woods burning and the fawn Bambi crying for his mother. It gave him nightmares for three years. Many years later, his four-year-old granddaughter brought him a *Bambi* video, and he didn't want to see it. To him it was frightening, and he was afraid his grandchild would have nightmares, too. It is a beautiful movie for some, but for someone like him it was horrible. Hahnemann tells us to behave as objective, unprejudiced observers. We homeopaths do not always do this.

Be an Objective Observer and Know What Is Normal

We cannot assume any similarity between our reactions and those of our patients.

Objectivity is often difficult. We see patients who have gone through incest, which is a very sensitive thing to discuss with patients. Some of you may understand what it is like. When you have experienced incest in your own life and then a patient tells you about incest and you see the patient's tears, what happens when you are not an objective prescriber? You prescribe for your own feelings. When you are very angry about incest, you may think your patient is angry, too. You will look for the rubric "Mind, Anger," expecting others to experience your feelings. To my astonishment, in my years of practice I have had patients tell me this was a beautiful experience in their lives. [*Some people actually find it erotic.*] I have also seen people in car accidents who started to laugh.

Try to find out what is normal *behavior in a certain situation and what is not, because we must prescribe on the strange, rare, and peculiar.*

When someone who is 20 years old likes to observe birds or flowers, this is normal. When a child five years old asks for a microscope because he likes to see an insect's tiny legs, what is this? Precocity. If a baby of six months old weeps because he is hungry, this is healthy. Do you prescribe *Pulsatilla*? No, you give him his milk. When a little child six or seven years of age is sitting at the table while his mother sets the table and starts to cry because he is very hungry, this is a symptom. He can see that food is coming, so this is strange. When someone is 82 years old, there is food on the table, and the person cries because of hunger, this is from childishness or weakness or possibly because they cannot see the food. The patient's age also may show what behavior is normal.

If we suffer the death of someone and we cry, is this normal? Yes, it is normal. If 10 years afterward we are still crying, we need a remedy because our energy is not strong enough to overcome this grief. To be a good homeopath, you have to know what health is, what normal is, what illness is, and what symptoms are important. In the beginning, my mistake was that I thought how I observed the world was normal. I learned, through helping patients, that my view is simply that—*mine*; it is not necessarily what is normal.

As we have said before, it is not what happens in somebody's life that matters but how he or she reacts to it. For example, a woman was in a fire in her car. There were flames, and she jumped out of her car. Normal or abnormal? [*Normal.*] She got out of the car, ran from it, and then said, "Gosh, I forgot my purse." She went back into the car, took her purse, opened it, took out the car key and locked the car, and then ran away. She was afraid someone would steal her car! This is not normal. It's interesting to see how people react during accidents.

Some years ago I was lecturing about something, and the fire alarm went off. I was in front of the class, and I had the most wonderful picture of the whole Materia Medica right in front of me by observing my colleagues. One person was astonished and could not move, one ran for the elevator, another one ran to keep someone else from getting on the elevator, one came back for his bag, one came back to take his *Kent's Repertory*, one looked terribly frightened, and one ran to the window to consider jumping. I stood and watched, so fascinated I couldn't move. Who had the healthiest reaction? Was I the healthiest for standing there and watching? No. This was the most wonderful lesson.

Try to be objective by keeping yourself out of the consultation. Though sometimes difficult, it is most important to simply watch what is going on.

When you are standing in front of a class, you see some people yawning, some people rubbing their stomachs, some looking interested, and some looking bored. We have to see where illness is and where health is. This is something that is lacking in both allopathic *and* homeopathic education. Rarely in our education are we taught the study of and differentiation between what is normal and what is not.

Psora Case 1—Followup

Six months later, this child has grown in height, is not answering as timidly, and sits more upright. The child says that 30 minutes after the remedy, he got a headache and stomachache. The same evening he got an earache. The next evening he started to perspire a lot and was soaked. One month later he got herpes on his lips. In one month, his sleep became profound and good. His mother said he had grown emotionally and did not weep as much. Four months ago his nose was blocked, and the next day his nose started to run and ran for six weeks, with a lot of discharge. For the past five days, he has had an earache and starts to weep again. He goes to school alone now. Before he got his remedy, his mother had to take him to school each day.

Did the remedy work? [*Definitely.*] Did it work in the correct way? Yes; he is taller, goes to school alone, and had an initial aggravation. He had a return of old symptoms and a discharge, with profuse sweating. (Aggravations must be followed by amelioration.) His sleep is better, and he is not weeping as much, has no cough, and has grown some. He has begun playing the guitar, which means he is more flexible and more creative. But now the earache is back, and he is crying again. Is the remedy still working? Who has suffered earaches? [*They're horrible.*] Yes. I repeated the remedy six months after the first dose. Why? A relapse of symptoms that were gone for six months. His weeping is back, so there were physical and emotional relapses.

When I know a remedy has worked beautifully and then relapses, I do not give a different potency right away. I have the proof that this potency worked; therefore, I do not see why I should change it.

His mother phoned about four weeks later.

Mother—How long do you think he has to have his earache after the remedy?

HH—What is happening?

Mother—His ear is still aching, and it's quite long after the remedy. I don't like for him to suffer this long.

I asked for the symptoms, and they were exactly the same as when I saw him here. No change. What does this mean to us? The second dose did not work, yet the first dose caused an aggravation, and then he was better. This situation means that he needs another potency. As a beginner when you do not trust yourself, you question the remedy. I know that the choice was right, so I changed the potency. This time I prescribed *Calcarea* 1M. Within 20 minutes, his earache was gone, and the weeping was gone. The next morning, he said to his mother, "Mom, how could it have been that I was always so weak? You know, I feel strong enough to go on the scouting holiday. I'd like to do it." The mother was happy because not only was his ear better but also he was maturing emotionally. He had never wanted to go away alone before.

When I went to the next seminar, I asked the homeopath why the boy wasn't in the seminar for a followup. He said, "Why? He has no symptoms anymore. He is fine. He has grown 15 centimeters (within six months after the remedy). You will not recognize him." In less than one year, he has practically no problems. What does this mean? His active psora is cured. The disturbance that made his life difficult had been cured. Why did *Calcarea* 200C do a good job and 1M complete it? Maybe the 1M would have been better in the beginning, but because of the weakness I did not want to give him this dose. Is he cured and happy for the rest of his life? No, he'll have his ups and downs, but what will come later?

What Can Happen Next

Schizophrenia, cancer, and suicide were in his family history. The syphilitic miasm is in his family history, and before he comes to latent psora, his vital force will bring forth syphilitic symptoms.

The miasms of a patient's ancestors will come out with signs and symptoms in the patient, showing that his miasmatic background is now active and has to be treated.

We must recognize the stage the patient is in. What might we see? At a certain moment, this patient could come back with skin problems, perhaps cracks in the corners of his mouth, a crack in his nose, a painful sore in his nose that he always picks at, or cracks in his heels. This will be a healthy way for the body to give the signal that another miasmatic picture is coming, something that is not psoric, which will require a different remedy. Our teaching today is about why this is a case of psora. This child protected himself, and the mother said he felt helpless. This is psoric behavior. With syphilis, there are different kinds of destruction. We can keep severe illnesses away from our patients by treating their miasms. This is the wonderful thing about homeopathy.

Questions From the Class

[*In looking at the strange, rare, and peculiar, why did you exclude the enuresis he had for so long?*]

When I saw him, it was gone. We did not need to treat it at this moment. What kind of miasm can have enuresis? All of them. How many remedies can have enuresis? All, as all can have headaches and pain in their limbs. These are clinical symptoms. Why would a psoric case have enuresis? Weakness of the sphincters. As soon as the bladder gets a little full, it has no strength. An easy case of enuresis can be gone in a few weeks. In a complicated case, such as a child with enuresis and epilepsy or diarrhea or sleeplessness, the *first and most important thing* for the vital force to cure is the *weakness.*

The body's vital force is responsible for curing the disturbance in the body.

If someone has epilepsy, stomach cramps, sleeplessness, and enuresis, what is the first thing you expect to happen after the remedy? He will sleep at night so his body can heal. Epilepsy is the most severe problem, but the body needs sleep to heal the other problems. An allopath tries to cure the epilepsy first, but we must cure the *patient.*

For example, if we treat a patient with migraines, some fear, some anxieties, and some digestion problems, what is the patient coming to us for? [*Migraines.*] Twice a week he has to lie down. What is he focused on? [*His migraines.*] After the remedy, we get a phone call that he is totally the same. As a beginning homeopath, you may doubt your remedy choice. However, when you see better color and more strength, you will know to keep "hands off" because he shows improvement. The patient is focused on his headaches—this is logical. The patient comes to us because he cannot find the solution for his problems. We are the professionals, and we have to be able to determine whether the remedy has a good reaction or not. In my first four years of homeopathy, I went up and down all the time. One day I would decide to quit completely, and another day when a patient was happy I was very pleased that I had chosen the right profession.

[*If this patient had grown, played the guitar, and become more confident but still put emphasis on small things like mice, would you have repeated the remedy then?*]

When someone is treated with *Calcarea* and the fear of mice is still there, what do we have to do? I can give you a simple case as an example. A very large woman came into my practice because of pain in her left shoulder (she had had it for five or six years) after a cow had kicked her. The wound healed quickly, but the pain remained. She cared for more than 100 cows twice a day (milking and feeding). Another complaint was urticaria. Every time she was in the sun, she had itching and burning. In the summer she did harvesting, and she would get ill from sitting on the tractor and being exposed to the sun. She also had an awful fear of mice. When she was in the stable with the cows and saw a little mouse, she would draw up her skirt, jump on the table, and scream about the mice. Her husband had to come for her. She sweated a lot, needed eggs, news reports were too upsetting for her, and she was constipated. Clearly she was in a *Calcarea* state.

So what do you think *Calcarea* would cure? The pain, the urticaria, or fear of mice? We have wonderful theories that tell us that first the mental symptoms will be cured, then the shoulder will be cured, then the skin. But in this woman's case, if her fear of mice remained, she could live forever with it. Another *Calcarea* woman (who also had fear of mice) made her living making clothes. If she saw a mouse while sitting at the sewing machine, she would remain frozen until someone came home to look for the mouse and try to find it. She could not do anything unless the whole house was searched for mice. She also had some headaches and joint pain. Where was she ill? [*In her mind.*] The first woman was ill in her body. We have to know what is the most prominent, dangerous, or threatening thing. That is what must be cured by the vital force.

Who in this room has no fear? To be a little fearful is healthy. One patient said she was on the 34th floor of an office building and had to step away from the windows because it made her dizzy. This is quite normal. Another patient was dizzy just standing on a step. This is abnormal. Sometimes we like to cure things in the beginning that do not need to be cured. If someone is dancing, do you have to cure this? Of course not. Know what is curable and what is important to cure.

[*If the fear of mice went away but her limiting problem was still there, then what would you do?*]

I would see how the case develops. When the remedy is doing something and there is no serious problem, I wait. Sometimes you will get aggravations (after the correct remedy) from a complaint the patient never had before, and you get anxious. A businessman was given *Nux vomica* by a homeopath and then went back after two months to tell her his energy was better after the remedy. "But give me another dose because now I do not feel so strong." The impatient homeopath prescribed another dose. Then the patient came back demanding yet *another* dose. Later I saw him, and he had a lot of sadness. He told me that he had been impotent since the fourth dose. He was depressed. I looked at the file then and saw the quick repetition of the remedy. Because he was not my patient, I did not prescribe anything at that moment. I wrote on his file that *Nux vomica* should never be given again and that it should be allowed to work its way out of his system.

Which of us could instruct the vital force how and when to work on a problem? My patients have taught me more than books. You learn so much in observing and trying to find the logical way of the vital force. Sometimes you can have an aggravation in a spot where you do not expect it. You are the expert. Think logically. With every new patient, you will see things you have never seen before.

[*With the boy this morning, is there anything you can see that might antidote his remedy?*]

I do not think you can antidote a remedy. I think the energy level of the patient can diminish, but this does not mean that he has antidoted his remedy. How long can a remedy work? The remedy acts in about 1/10 of a second and can continue to act for as long as the energy of the patient can sustain improvement in health. I'd like to explain what I see about energy. Remember the game dominoes? When they are placed upright in a long row, even a row many miles long, one touch can cause all the dominoes to fall in sequence the whole way. If you line up 10 boxes of dominoes, it takes one stimulus, (the touch) to start the falling but the falling can continue as long as there are dominoes. If an outside energy is strong enough to stop the dominoes somewhere along the way, such as sticking one's finger in the way, it stops the reaction (the falling), but it has not touched the stimulus. Can a child antidote the stimulus? No; but he can disturb the result. When you touch the energy level of the patient with a remedy, can you undo the touch? No, but you can interfere with the continued reaction by drinking lots of coffee because the coffee artificially stimulates your adrenal glands, giving you the sensation that you have more energy. Consequently, you use more energy than you have naturally and deplete your vital energy, which is needed for healing. I think you can disturb the patient's energy needed for healing, just as too great a stress can interfere with continued healing, causing a relapse, but you cannot antidote the remedy.

[*Can you repeat a remedy every time you see a relapse?*] You would repeat if it is a true relapse and if the patient is going back to his less healthy state. Usually a relapse does not take him as far back as in the beginning of the case. Cure never occurs in a straight line; it is always a wavy line. Is there anybody in the world who remains forever in a steady line of energy and health? No, never. There are two possibilities: You move up in a wavy line or down in a wavy line. When the energy of a patient stands still and does not improve anymore or when there are signs of a true relapse, you give the remedy again and it will work. Be as logical as you can be. As soon as you make rules, you will find the patient who is the exception.

Psora Case 2: Boy With Encopresis and Behavior Problems

This child was abandoned by his parents. He is seven years old and lives in a children's home where his father visits him perhaps once every six months. The father comes to go walking on a Sunday and takes the boy back to the home at 4:00 P.M. The child hasn't seen his mother for years.

He still always expects his mother, but only the father comes and only occasionally. Can you imagine what it is like for him waiting every week for his mother to come? A foster family had the idealistic idea to care for him on weekends and holidays and show him some love and normal family life, but the care was so difficult (the child behaved so badly) that they went to psychologists for advice on how to handle him. At one point they said, "We will not take him anymore." They were fed up. How do you imagine the child feels now? Again, abandoned. A friend of this foster family is a homeopath, who suggested that the foster mother try homeopathy, so the foster mother came with the child to our practice.

Video Presentation and Case Description

The following discussion was captured as it occurred during a video presentation and case description by Henny Heudens. Student questions and comments appear in brackets. In the interview portions, "HH" indicates a question or comment by Henny, and "P" indicates the patient's comment or response.

The boy is looking at his foster mother. He is very blonde. I explain to him that there are colleagues upstairs looking at him on video. I ask him to talk louder so people can hear his voice, but he does not do it. What do you see so far? [*He's shy.*] He covers his face with his hands, flushes, and pulls away from the camera. This is a boy who stole my heart. I feel a lot of pity when I hear the report of a bad boy doing a lot of bad things. I see a sweet, poor boy who has gone through a lot of misery in his life. What kind of a remedy do we need? [*Psoric.*] Yes, we know immediately it has to be psoric. I ask what he likes most in the whole world. He says, "Mud. I like to play in the mud, and I like to make things with mud—pour water in the dirt and make pigs." I ask what else he likes to play with, and he leans back looking at the sky. Is he able to answer? Is he clever or not? [*Yes.*] How do you know? [*You can see it in his eyes.*] I ask this question so he will talk with me.

Then I ask him another question. "If you could choose something in the world you'd like the most, what would you choose?" He is looking up in the air, and then you see in his eyes that he has quit thinking. These are questions psychologists have probably already asked him a lot. The mother says to him, "Go on, you know. You know what you have to tell. Again you start to play your tricks!" What happens with the boy after such a remark? [*He pulls away.*] The foster mother is fed up with him. We hear this in her remark. She is so frustrated she even shows it on video in public. I see that the child looks humiliated. I feel sorry for the child. After the mother pushed him to speak, he answers automatically.

HH—What do you like to play with?
P—Legos.
Mother—He builds houses and he plays with cars.
HH—Do you break them when you play with them?
P—Sometimes.
HH—Why do you break them?
P—Sometimes by accident.
HH (to the mother)—Can you describe how he plays?
Mother—He is always outside. He is busy.

Watch the relationship between them. Is there a possibility at this time for them to come together? [*No.*] We see many mothers in our practice, and we watch how they behave. Most touch their children, and when you ask the child a difficult question, they try to put an arm around the child or give him some encouragement. They may repeat the question softly to help the child understand. Here, there is no help from the foster mother. I feel the child is really alone. What is the child doing now? He is flushing a lot again, and he is hanging over my desk. He likes me, as I like him.

Until now, what do we have? [*Psora—flushing, timidity, loneliness.*] Do we see grief or anger yet? No, not a lot. We hear about a child who likes to play outside. What more do we observe in him? It sometimes helps to watch what is happening on the video without sound. [*He is fidgeting, restless.*] Restless to the extent that it is unusual? No, not extraordinarily. [*He is a very sensitive child.*] Imagine you are seven years old. Your parents abandon you, and you finally get a "weekend mother" who abandons you. What would his reaction be? I'm sure that one or two of you have experienced this situation. Some children will think there is something wrong with them, and what is their reaction to that feeling? They can behave badly to prove there is something wrong with them, or they can be depressed. They will withdraw—not learning, not studying, and perhaps not playing. This is not the case with this boy; he enjoys playing.

What is another way of reacting to the feeling that you have been abandoned? [*Trying to please someone, clinging to them.*] Yes, wanting people to constantly tell you they love you. Why are there these different reactions to the same situation? Because of the differences in our constitutions. How will a syphilitic person react? [*Violently.*] How? [*Killing a pet, breaking something, hitting someone.*] That is why I asked how he plays with his toys. If he hits his sister in the head, this might be syphilitic, but until now we see psora in this boy. To try to find some argument for other miasms instead of psora, I ask him when he gets angry. "When I don't get what I want." He says he isn't afraid of any of the things I ask him about. He does not remember about when he was small. The mother then says that he has mentioned being afraid of the dark. She tells him he does not remember a lot of things.

I ask the foster mother to tell me the good things about him. Now his face looks happy; he agrees with what she is telling. She says he is concerned about her. "When we're walking outside in the fields, he takes away the plants that might hurt me (stinging nettle)."

How many of you have children, and have any of yours done this for you? I have lovely children, but I had to do this for them. This boy, seven years old, spreads the plants so his mother can walk without being hurt. This is appreciation—love and caring for his foster mother who does not even show much attachment to him. You see how happy he is to tell this. His contact with me is very good. Can you imagine him being a bad boy?

What is the problem according to his foster mother? "He makes stool during the day in his pants, and he walks around all day until someone says something. He never tells that he has done it; other people in the family have to smell it." The mother told me that one day she tried not to react to see how long he would keep the stool in his pants; he left it until his bath in the evening. Do you think there is something wrong with his anus? [*No.*] Why not? [*Because if there was something wrong with his anus, he would go clean himself or say something.*] Yes. He also wets his bed, which is not normal, but many other children do it at this age. Stool in his pants is not very common at this age. He does this at the children's home, and they have given him pampers. This is why the mother is so fed up with him. He does this every day for all bowel movements. They did toilet training, trying to make him sit on the toilet until he made stool, and he would not wipe his bottom even when he defecated. The only time he does not make stool in his pants is when his father comes to take him out on the weekend. Every weekend he talks about when his father will come. He always asks whether his father knows where to find him.

At the foster home, there are two other children in the family, a boy and girl.

HH—How does he behave with them?

Mother—He almost always quarrels with the boy, but not with the little sister whom he protects.

When the foster brother takes something away from the little girl, this boy protects the girl. The two get along very well, building castles, and so forth. When they come home, they are dirty from head to foot and have had a wonderful time.

HH—How does he sleep?

Mother—Very well.

Why am I interested to know about the sleep of a child with emotional disturbances? You might expect nightmares or bad dreams after being abandoned. He dreams about his father and about his birth parents, dreams that he is with them and playing with them.

HH—(I ask again) "What is your wish in life if you could have anything we could give you?

P—My parents.

I ask him about crying, but his mother answers instead.

Mother—He cries a lot when he hurts himself, even a little. He wants to be caressed. He takes all the attention I can give. I can tell our little girl that it's OK when she hurts herself, but not with him. Now I don't do it anymore. I make him go play.

The mother feels he is cheating her, weeping all day long about a small wound, trying to get all her attention. She said he finds her weak spots. I ask how he reacts to music? She answers that there is nothing special, just like all the other children.

HH—How is he in school?

Mother—A big problem. He does not work; cannot calculate, read, or write; and always causes problems in class. Whenever he gets attention, he wants more. It is never enough.

She has stopped giving him more attention. She said that when the relationship was better before, she could speak with him, and she had the feeling he felt guilty about not being with his parents. He felt it was his fault. What miasm do we see? [*Psora.*] Yes. He has a physical allergy to milk. He cannot digest it. He has asthmatic breathing and uses inhalers. When I ask him about food, see how he looks at his foster mother. Does he understand what she is saying? He is trying to understand.

HH—What does he like to eat?

Mother—Pastry, meat, ice cream, lemons, cucumbers, pancakes; he has aversion to tortellini and fish, and he hates the bread I bake myself.

I ask him and the mother how his behavior is toward animals, and the mother says he loves animals.

HH—What kind of animals do you like?

P—Pigs.

This is a strange answer. The mother says they call him "our pig" because he loves pigs so much, and he is always playing in the mud. "We call him 'Piggy.'" Until now we need a psoric remedy who likes ice cream a lot, and one who likes to play outside.

Psora Case 2—Analysis

What are the characteristics we need to prescribe a remedy for this boy?

[*Forsaken, desire for company.*] Which of you would feel forsaken if you were this child? Everyone. Imagine being seven years old. Do you like company? You want someone to play with when you're seven years old, not being mature enough to do things alone. When a child of seven years of age likes to be alone, this would be a characteristic. With this boy, wanting to be cared for is not a symptom. If you prescribe on this, you will not find his remedy.

[*What I find unusual—if he wants to be loved—is that he leaves stool in his pants, which drives people away.*] Yes, this is a symptom. Stool in his pants, which every remedy can have, although some remedy states would not like it. This is the way he expresses his personal feelings. [*I find this unusual since he's so sensitive.*] Yes, he is very sensitive. Is being sensitive a symptom? No, we all need to be sensitive, but when we are oversensitive this is a symptom, just as it is a symptom when one is not sensitive at all. In his situation, is he oversensitive, not sensitive enough, or quite normal? [*Caring for the mother so well shows his oversensitivity.*] Yes, we all know that our own children do not do this. He is not sensitive about his own stool, but he is sensitive to the problems of others. It is characteristic for the boy that he is sensitive to his mother's suffering and that he loves pigs. Where do we see more sensitivity? [*The way he takes care of the little girl.*] Why does he react to her differently from the eight-year-old boy? [*Because he can take care of her.*] Yes, he is very protective and helps her.

He loves animals, and he always sleeps with toy animals in his bed. What does he love the most? [*Pigs.*] Do we have "loves pigs" in the Materia Medica? [*No.*] But there are remedies known to be helpful for pigs and horses if the animal's behavior and symptom picture is similar to the symptoms of the remedy. Do we have a remedy that loves pigs? It would be nice. (He is sliding down in his chair so I have to adjust the video here.) His mother says he lies and steals a lot. She says she does not think she can keep him in her home any longer because of the stealing and because of the stool. She says, "It is too much."

In what way does he like pigs? He likes the mud. This is a characteristic of the boy. What else happens with him? [*I would not expect him to have so much social charm because of the abandonment. I think some children would be more withdrawn.*] Either more withdrawn or more violent. He does not react violently, and he does not overdo as in sycotic behavior. He is behaving shyly with guilty feelings. This is how psora presents. We need a psoric remedy that makes stool in pants, but every remedy can do this. He does not care about it. He likes mud, and so mud is in his pants. It does not bother him at all. For him it is no problem at all, but it is a problem for his mother.

Could this be a *Calcarea carbonica* boy? [*He has no fears or anxieties.*] [*Leaving the stool in his pants all day is a serious mental disturbance, so it has gone to the mental sphere.*] Yes, if he were *Calcarea* and went to school all day and people noticed the smell of stool on him, he would not like others having a bad opinion about him. We need a remedy for someone who does not care what others think.

This is a clear *Sulphur* case. What other symptoms do you see in this child that are clearly *Sulphur*?

- Loves to play and get dirty all day without mentioning it
- Likes to play in the mud
- Flushes in the face
- Desires fresh air, likes to play outside
- Prefers sweets, ice cream
- Is a caretaker (*Sulphur* is a caretaker for weaker ones and for family members.)

Why is he waiting for his father every weekend, even when his logic tells him his father abandoned him? Why does he dream about his family instead of having nightmares? Because *Sulphur* has only one care and one fear, and that is that something will happen to his family. He is sensitive toward his mother and his little sister. Why does he love pigs? They are muddy, dirty animals. *Sulphur* thinks things that are dirty are nice.

What else is a *Sulphur* symptom? [*Not paying attention at school, being bored, daydreaming.*] Not concentrating on things he is not interested in. This is a *Sulphur* symptom. He made contact with the foster mother here on the video; he reached out to her. He weeps easily, and this is not well known for *Sulphur*, but it is bold in *Kent's Repertory* under **MIND; WEEPING**. Of course, any remedy can weep. Aversion to fish, desires meat, and milk aggravates are all *Sulphur* symptoms.

I took this case with my colleagues watching upstairs. When we analyzed the case, they expected me to give the child an extraordinary remedy. I was astonished. They had arguments for small remedies. I gave him *Sulphur.* I will show you the followup. After this consultation, I had a long letter from the foster mother. She sent a psychological description of the illness of the child, with remarks from the psychologist of how there is no cure for this child, how difficult his life will be, and how he will become a criminal with no conscience. The mother sent me this psychological evaluation one week after the remedy. She felt better now that she had this analysis of him, because in her mind it allowed her to give up on him. She then felt it would be all right to abandon this child since he could not be helped. I asked the mother to bring the child back again in six months. She abandoned him for the first month after the remedy in that she did not get him from the children's home on weekends.

Psora Case 2—Followup

At this six-month followup the foster mother and boy are sitting together and holding hands, and she is looking at him. She is caring for him. Her expression toward him is now one of love. We are approaching the holidays, and the mother says that he got a headache just before this visit. Often children get headaches or sleeplessness before the holidays from expectations of what is coming. The mother says that it is cozy at home now. He comes for a weekend every three weeks, and he visits every Sunday. He'll be home with them for the Christmas holidays. The mother has changed. She says it is a lot better with him in school "*because he has a new teacher.*"

We often hear these explanations from our patients after a homeopathic remedy, because after their remedy they are able to react in the world in ways that allow them to begin to get the things that they need, the things that are good for them, that are healthy for them.

He has not stolen anymore.

How is he now, six months after the remedy? Do you feel so much pity for him? No, you can tell he feels better. He says now he'd like to be with his foster family (he calls them "Dad" and "Mom" for the first time). He has adopted them now.

HH—How about your real father and mother?

P—They don't visit me, so this is my mother.

This means he has overcome the problem of abandonment.

HH—With whom do you like to play?

P—With my brother and sister.

All three are now a family.

HH—How is he doing in school?

Mother—He is doing reasonably well. He is starting to read and calculate. His tests are not extraordinary, but they are much better than before.

HH—How about his stool?

Mother—Oh, that; it's gone.

HH—If I could do magic for you and give you anything in the world, what is your wish?

P—To get a real pig.

For Christmas, he got a piggy bank. I asked about his anger, and the mother said there is more sadness than anger. In his situation, this is a normal emotion that is now coming out.

At the end of the interview, the mother says that she and her husband (six months after the remedy) are discussing adopting the boy. What will this mean for the child, and why does this happen? The mother looks satisfied now. Her voice is soft now; she loves the boy. It's as if we gave a remedy to the mother. This is the wonderful thing in homeopathy. You treat one person in the family, and then other family members feel better because the tension is gone, so in treating one person the whole family gets better. Old-fashioned *Sulphur* did the trick, a remedy that is sometimes not thought of today because it is not an exotic remedy. My experience is that we can help most of our patients with the old-fashioned remedies. There are many remedies being proven today that were not known or proven in Hahnemann's day, but do not forget these old-fashioned, well-proven remedies that have been used successfully for 200 years.

We all see a lot of cases similar to the one we have just discussed, where we need to treat children born into families with parents who have left them to the care of others. What is the common problem for these children? [*Anger, depression, guilt, confusion, low self-esteem, behavior disorders.*] Yes, I think the schools are filled with these children. They act out in school, and the parents are told that these children have attention deficit-hyperactive disorder (ADHD). When this label is put on children, they are considered essentially hopeless allopathically. Special schools and special teachers with psychological training help them deal with their problems, but allopathically there is little that can be done to restore health in these children.

Everywhere in the world, children and parents suffer in this situation. Without homeopathy, attention deficit or hyperactive children can be so difficult to deal with that they cannot develop loving relationships or positive emotions. Without the example of a stable family, these poor children often grow up unable to make a stable family of their own. Some children stay with the grandparents. Some children are abandoned and are in foster care. Foster parents invite these children into their homes for the weekends and holidays to give the children love and some semblance of normal family life. Sometimes these children are successfully integrated into the foster family, but so often we see suffering in the foster parents because they cannot cope with the situation. They want to help and are idealistic in their desire to make a difference in the lives of these children, but often they suffer with sorrow and fear and disappointment because the children are so ill and they are unable to help them.

CHAPTER 2

Syphilis and the Syphilitic Miasm

Syphilis is a miasm and a disease. In homeopathy, unless we are treating a patient with active syphilis, we generally speak not of the disease itself, but of the result of the disease having been suppressed in the past and now showing itself as a tendency toward illness in a person or in a family. What we see is an inherited vulnerability. When I use the words "syphilis" and "syphilitic" in this discussion, I mean the miasm unless otherwise stated.

The syphilitic miasm has **destructive tendencies**; it may **destroy tissue**. A patient can be restored to health only when the miasms in the patient are inactive or latent. If the symptoms of a patient with a syphilitic background are suppressed rather than cured, a deeper, more serious disease may emerge from the "miasm pot." For this reason, we must know the miasmatic history of our patients.

In Hahnemann's time, when someone had the disease of syphilis, mercury was applied to the syphilitic chancre (and sometimes given internally) to remove the chancre, and often the chancre went away. Did the illness go away? No. Think again about the example we have all heard in our homeopathic training: if someone is bitten on the arm or leg by a poisonous snake and the arm or leg is then cut off, is the person cured? The location of the bite is gone, but is the poison out of the body? No. It has traveled throughout the body. It is the same with the disease of syphilis. It spreads throughout the organism. It is the same with vaccinations. If someone is vaccinated on the arm, the person may get a little ulcer (or sometimes react more strongly). Three weeks later, a cough or epilepsy might develop. Something that happens locally may have an effect on the entire organism. This is what happens with the disease of syphilis.

What does the real syphilitic disease look like? We have all seen it in the third stage, probably without knowing it was the disease of syphilis. For example, we may see dullness, an inability to express emotions, depression, or physical disturbances. At the end, the disease of syphilis breaks down the whole body, even after treatment with modern allopathy. In Hahnemann's time, allopaths tried to remove the syphilitic chancre locally. However,

Hahnemann discovered that the children and even the grandchildren of people thus treated—that is, whose syphilitic disease symptoms had been suppressed—inherited the dreadful effects of the disease of syphilis.

Although psora was spread through simple touch and its miasmatic symptoms are easily recognizable as the result of psora's universal influence in all of humanity, this was not true of the chronic influence of syphilis. Rather than the simple innocence of touch, the spread of the disease syphilis required sexual contact with someone who was already infected with the syphilitic disease. This required the use of will: One had to choose to act in a certain way. Often accompanying the severity of the disease of syphilis was a sense of wickedness or corruption and the desire to hide its evidence.

Today, a patient's miasms can be discerned from the symptoms in the person and in her or his family history, but few of us can know whether someone's father or grandfather had the disease of syphilis, because people usually do not speak openly about it. We do not tell our children when we contract the disease of syphilis. It is kept hidden—a disease that is "unacceptable" to society. Within the syphilitic miasm picture is the issue of hiding. The patient wants to hide the fact that he has or had syphilis. It is not hiding due to the shyness or sense of shame that we find in psora. It is being secretive in many ways, and we will see many examples in our syphilitic patients of keeping secrets, not wanting us to know their secrets. We will also see that the symptoms of syphilitic miasm are often hidden beneath the surface, destroying beneath the surface

In case taking, always take the history of the parents and grandparents as well, so that you know the weaknesses of the families on both sides. Of the patient's symptoms, look for the progression of illness as it developed from birth into later life. In some cases, the patient's current symptoms may run throughout the case from pre-birth—from somewhere in the family background, all the way to the present time. When the syphilitic miasm is in a case, psora is there already, so we have a psoric/syphilitic case. When two miasms are combined, cases are more difficult; we have to treat each miasm.

Mental and Emotional Symptoms and Expressions of the Syphilitic Miasm

Dullness	Aggression
Emptiness	Violence

Silence	Rage
Closed	Danger
Secrecy	Feelings of being threatened
No connection	Feelings of being attacked
Isolation	Feelings of being surrounded by enemies
Suspicion	Misery
Fear of others	Perversion
Killing	Destruction
Knives	Suicide

What are the signs and symptoms of the syphilitic miasm? **Dullness** is a strong symptom. Syphilitic patients with this dullness do not comprehend things. We may tell syphilis something 10 or more times, and he will say, "Okay." But when we ask him about it later, he does not remember. Syphilitic children have problems in school because of this dullness. What we often see in psoric children is that they **try hard** to do their best. Often this is compensation, so other people will not see that they are weak. But dull, syphilitic children sit there with **expressionless**, **empty faces**. They strive to do well in school, but there is **emptiness** in their eyes. They cannot concentrate and have trouble absorbing what they read. The inability to concentrate and the dullness make it hard for them to learn mathematics, which is a very strong symptom in children with the syphilitic miasm.

With the syphilitic miasm, there is a kind of **silence**. Some syphilitic patients cannot tell us very much. While psoric patients may spend hours talking, we have to pull words out of a syphilitic patient. If she tells only some superficial things or if she does not tell enough, this is a sign of the syphilitic miasm. Syphilitic children and adults are mostly silent, with little ability to express their thoughts and feelings. They are **"closed"** and hold in their feelings. There is even a **barrier** within the syphilitic person between her own feelings and her mind. In her syphilitic state she is just not very bright about knowing or telling her sensations and feelings. This is not a criticism or judgement, but rather a clue that you will notice during case taking.

Some women fall in love with silent, syphilitic men. They have the impression that these men are silent because they are wise. After three years of marriage, these women discover that this silence stems not from wisdom but from emptiness—there is nothing inside. The syphilitic miasm may give the impression of listening, but syphilitic people do not react because there is **no connection** to their feelings and therefore little to express. They are not in touch with their own feelings. The dullness in a syphilitic person's facial expression could be mistaken for shyness. Some women tell me that their husbands sit staring at the television, not even following the program. "He only sits there and stares." This could be a sign of syphilis. Wives may say about their husbands, "It is so boring to be married to him." Syphilitic patients have this kind of dullness in the mind, as opposed to the weakness of the psoric person.

Syphilis has fears but not the fears of psora, who does not feel strong enough to handle a situation. Syphilis has a special **fear of other people**. He does not trust other people because he believes others could kill him. This **mistrust** of people also includes a lack of trust in himself. He knows that these possibilities for **killing** are within him as well. When syphilis walks down the street, he may feel that somebody is following him, so he constantly looks behind. He believes someone could be there who might have a knife or a gun and want to kill him. He is suspicious. There is something in him that fears other people. While psora feels poor and fears that someone will take something from her, syphilis fears being killed. From syphilis we hear many expressions around the idea of danger.

The idea of not trusting himself also means that even when syphilis has washed his hands, he has to wash them again because they may not be clean enough. This is one symptom of the remedy *Syphilinum.* The Materia Medica notes that *Syphilinum* does not trust himself. For example, when he locks the door, he is unsure that he has done it so he has to check it again. Syphilis also may be very **inflexible** or have fixed ideas. When something is in his mind, he cannot let go of it. His behavior may become compulsive. Syphilis is fastidious because of **danger** but not fastidious in the psoric way. Psora wants the good opinion of others and therefore chooses to be fastidious to look good for others. Syphilis is fastidious because he feels **threatened** or is simply inflexible about an idea. Syphilis feels that germs could kill him. He may feel a need to bathe, brush his teeth, or change his clothes many times a day.

Syphilis experiences life as dangerous. One wonderful sunny day, a patient came into my consulting room with an umbrella. It is strange to see somebody with an umbrella when it does not look like rain, so I said, "Oh, do you think it will rain today?" He told me that he always carries an umbrella. "I carry it always a little forward so that if someone seems dangerous to me I can stab him." In *Kent's Repertory*, there is the rubric **MIND; DELUSIONS;** ***shoot, tries to, with a cane.*** One remedy, *Mercurius.* My patient could not carry a knife or gun legally so he carried an umbrella instead. If syphilis wants to travel, what does he take with him? A gun? A knife? Mace?

A hypothetical scenario: Syphilis is walking down the street. She is very weak after having the flu and having been treated with antibiotics. She hears someone behind her. She has a knife in her pocket, and her hand is on the knife because she knows that someone is behind her. She is **suspicious.** She turns and cuts the person with no provocation. Syphilis may punch someone in the face with no provocation because of her state of alarm. She fights first because of her fear of danger.

Syphilis has a strong **fear of being killed** and a fear of knives. When syphilis sees a knife, something awful happens to her. On seeing the knife, she thinks that she has to stab and kill herself or someone else. Syphilitics are lovely people, and unless she revealed such thoughts in a homeopathic consultation, we would never know of her struggle. She gets these thoughts because one of her ancestors had syphilis (the disease) and it was suppressed. Now she has an awful fear of knives and does not know why.

Syphilitic people may even fear killing their own children. One of my patients was afraid that he would kill his baby with a knife. He was **terrified** that he would hurt his child. He felt awful. He could not talk about it with his wife, but he told me about it during the consultation because it was so troubling to him. After *Hyoscyamus,* the thought of hurting his child went away.

Normal parenting includes the desire to protect our children and give them a better life than we had because we love them. Syphilitic parents want this too, but along with love for their children may come the sudden thought that they have to take a knife and kill them. One of my patients would wake up in the night with a strong urge to kill her children. She was cured with the syphilitic remedy *Mercurius,* which has a feeling that she might kill someone.

Murderous thoughts sometimes occur in women who suffer from postpartum depression. In the past, these poor, ill women often were sent to an asylum, and their babies were taken away because the babies were in danger. Had these women received a homeopathic remedy, their suffering would have been relieved and they could have overcome their emotional illness without the loss of their children and incarceration in asylums.

We know how deeply emotionally ill people suffer. They may be very nice people, yet they suffer from a difficult internal struggle. At a certain moment, a syphilitic person may kill. It is known that some people who take certain antidepressants develop the **inclination to kill** other people. These are syphilitic individuals. The antidepressant touches their syphilitic miasm, not by curing it but by suppressing their syphilitic depression. When their symptoms re-emerge more strongly after suppression, these individuals may feel that they have to kill somebody. Nothing will quiet the syphilitic heritage except homeopathy.

Miasmatically, **aggression** and all sorts of destruction are syphilitic. Most violent crime is syphilitic. Syphilis likes violence, horror movies, guns, shooting, and killing. Watching **torture** and killing in movies, enjoying these films, and creating these films are symptomatic of the syphilitic miasm. Psora's reaction to violent films is to hide from them, run away, or cover her eyes, but syphilis enjoys them. Syphilis will watch closely to learn things he can use to protect himself. Syphilis also likes to read about violence.

When we are determining degrees of illness in the mind of a syphilitic person, we look for an increase in the destructiveness of her expressions as the severity of her disease increases. First we see hate, then violence, then the desire to kill, and then the actual killing, as the illness progresses within the organism. In the same way, when a severely ill, severely syphilitic patient begins to get better, her syphilitic expressions will be less and less destructive in quality, reflecting her improvement. With all symptoms, there are degrees of deepening pathology, but the pathology is not always so obvious. Sometimes pathology is masked in politeness. Someone may tell you in a polite, polished manner, "I am so sorry, but I have to kill you." Although syphilitic, the person has learned how to formulate conversation so that the feelings are not so obvious.

Professions and Behaviors

A person's profession can tell a lot about his inner state. Syphilitic individuals may choose professions where they can use a knife to do something constructive, creative, or even healing rather than killing. Consider a syphilitic person's career choice to be a chef. He can spend his energy chopping things. Even better, he could be a butcher and use the knife to **cut with power and force** at the same time. Many butchers are syphilitic. A syphilitic person who has more money and more education might become a surgeon. Don't forget that we all have miasms, which need expression, but not all methods of expression have to be harmful.

Imagine a person who is able to execute a fellow human being or carry out any form of the death penalty. In France a famous person executed more than 1,500 people on the guillotine. What might he have been feeling? It is difficult for some of us to imagine how anyone could do this job. I can only understand that he must be a syphilitic person. Could psora have such a profession? Impossible. Psora would never be able to sleep. Psora feels guilty after killing an insect.

How about postal workers who use guns against those who offend them? What about people who rob banks? A bank robber's typical scenario consists of first stealing a car and changing its license tag or paint. Then she puts on a black mask, "hiding her secret," takes a knife, a gun, or a bomb, and with full knowledge, takes money, kills people, or destroys the bank. When does she do this? In recent times, she'd steal during the day when there is more money in the bank, but in earlier times banks were robbed during the night—the syphilitic miasm is active in the night. She can kill without guilt. After the syphilitic criminal is sent to prison for 10 years, she may perfect her criminality, and when she comes out of prison, she is able to do more harm than before. I am not a politician, but I know that imprisonment cannot help this person. Perhaps the combination of prison and homeopathy might help her. After so many years of homeopathic practice, I can recognize a certain look in some people's faces and in their eyes that tells me that a simple, small offense against them may cause them to react in a big way. They may react with **extreme anger from a small provocation**—a syphilitic reaction.

Because syphilis likes to **hide**, he might be happy working in the secret service, spying for the state or for another country. This is syphilitic—always hiding, being totally capable of hiding in this position for 20 to 30 years, without even his wife knowing.

A policeman may be syphilitic. He might like to send people to prison or beat them, which shows the syphilitic miasm. However, I treat some policemen with psoric symptoms. Psora might want to be a policeman to show strength. To know the miasm, we have to know why he is a policeman.

Always ask "why" about a symptom—what is underneath a symptom. Why does a patient need this or that symptom?

It could be that the patient chooses a profession to face a fear or to experience his feelings in a safe environment. We must consider whether the patient's outward behavior is a reflection of his deep feelings or is a compensation for those feelings. We must treat the underlying feelings. In some cases, we can discover the patient's deeper feelings and his most natural personality by asking questions regarding his youth. Because his childhood is somewhat removed from his current circumstances, he may be more able to describe this early period of his life without editing his feelings.

After surgery, some patients do not come out of anesthesia well. Some are wild and violent, some cry, some pick at the bedclothes or try to get out of the restraints, and some just lie there and do nothing. Some sweet old ladies swear like troopers when they are not yet fully conscious. We are all unique, and when we do not have control of our minds, we do what is natural. The sweet old lady who was well behaved before the operation but who comes out swearing is syphilitic. After a sudden shock, our weaknesses are exposed.

Dreams are important because the real personality comes forth during these states when we are not guarding our fears and frailties. What is expressed just after waking is similar to what happens post-anesthesia. I hear histories from patients who tell me what goes on in their minds for the first few seconds after they wake up in the morning. We can see the miasms in these waking feelings and expressions.

Syphilis may feel that a **power is attacking her body** and destroying it. She may feel that something is creeping into her mouth and eating her intestines or that something is creeping into her anus or her vagina. She feels there is some force trying to destroy her. She may **fear germs** (as may psora), but the fear seen in syphilis shows some malevolent intention.

It is interesting to study the experiences people have with alcohol and other drugs. After taking pot, hashish, or LSD, a person might tell me that he wanted to commit suicide or jump from a tower. These "I don't want to live anymore" responses are strong syphilitic reactions. I also see young people who have had a bad LSD trip in which people are killing them or knocking them down; they may even think they are dead. This is the syphilitic expression.

How does syphilis react to an injustice done to him? He feels **rage** (growling is syphilitic) and may wait for a chance to seek revenge. He nurtures his feelings of revenge. When enraged, he is capable of smashing things, striking out, or hurting someone with a weapon or other object. He knows that he is even capable of killing. But the syphilitic miasm may dull the feelings so much that syphilis becomes a "cool" killer, killing without feeling. Holding a grudge is syphilitic. *Nitric acid* is a wonderful picture of this. The remedy *Nitric acid* is perhaps 80 percent syphilitic. Syphilitic patients deal with fear by attacking to protect themselves.

When syphilis feels sadness or grief, she holds it back and does not show it. When asked what is wrong, she will not say, cannot say. She **keeps it inside** where it simmers and **eats at her**. She isolates herself from other people, broods, and considers suicide. The grief cannot get out. She may actually commit suicide. The desire for death is a syphilitic expression. The person who kills herself after losing a loved one is syphilitic. We may hear of the quiet neighbor who never complained about anything and suddenly commits suicide—although no one was aware that anything was wrong because she never talked about it. Or we may hear that a neighbor, who was always so polite, suddenly took a gun and shot her entire family. People say how quiet and nice she was. When syphilis feels that **everybody is her enemy**, this may become too much to bear, and she may kill herself and sometimes others as well. Syphilis has delusions of being persecuted. She **hides her feelings** from her family and her neighbors, and out of this suppression may come **unexpected violent actions**, even political uprisings and anarchism.

When syphilis experiences an event he cannot digest emotionally, he may develop a **hatred** for it. He does not want to be touched by it. The general idea is that syphilis can hate. **Hate** is always found in syphilis. He hates his life, his neighbors, his food, and his environment. He uses the word "hate" a lot. When one mother told me she hated her daughter right in front of her daughter, it bothered me very much. But this can be the feeling of syphilis. Syphilis often describes things as "**rotten**." We may hear "I have a rotten personality" or "My life is rotten."

Misery is syphilitic. Syphilitic patients may be withdrawn, not making contact, not smiling. They project darkness. There is depression, apathy, and lack of connection. Once, while dining in a restaurant, I observed a couple who never looked at each other during the entire meal. They sat across from each other looking in all directions except into the face of the other. This is an example of the syphilitic lack of connection. Syphilis is often **disconnected** even within himself, as in schizophrenia—disconnected and **isolated**—as if he has been cut off from others, is on an island, and cannot find the "bridge" to another person. Every connection is broken. Syphilis may purposefully "cut" his connections, even breaking relationships with his family. There is this kind of destruction and indifference to protect himself from painful feelings. Syphilis is worse from touch. **Consolation aggravates** him—this is definitely syphilitic. He does not want touch, caresses, or kisses. Affection makes him feel worse.

If someone is in the waiting room with a syphilitic patient, that someone may get depressed just from being with syphilis. Syphilis may be dressed in dark brown, dark gray, or black. In the consulting room with the syphilitic patient, the homeopath mostly feels no contact, no connection, no vibrations. It may feel as if you are watching a film. There is a cold expression in the eyes, a lack of liveliness.

When syphilis buys a car, it will be a fast one because she likes to use her energy in a **dangerous** way, risking her life not so much for the thrill of it, but because she does not value life. Being inward and not finding it easy to show herself, she may show off her speedy car and use it to do dangerous things. One of my syphilitic patients did not care about his life, so he would cross the highway without looking. If someone hit him his life would be finished, and he did not care.

A syphilitic party might involve drinking, aggression, Russian roulette, perverted sex, shouting, and fighting. Syphilitic individuals may play dangerous games. I sense the syphilitic miasm in men whose way is macho—they like to fight, and their actions and intentions, indeed their lives, can be violent. They may buy motorcycles and wear leather with spikes. They may take risks by driving fast and taking curves too fast—engaging in risky behavior to be mean, not just for the excitement. Syphilis avoids the generally harmless excitements of sycosis or tuberculosis. It is the danger he likes. Some "accidents" in which people are killed are actually hidden homicides or suicides.

Biting, **cutting**, or scratching oneself to inflict pain is syphilitic. One may scratch or pick his skin from nervousness, but biting one's own flesh is very syphilitic. **Self-mutilation** and body piercing may indicate the presence of the syphilitic miasm. I have asked young people why they pierce themselves. Psora does it to be accepted. Sycosis does it to show off and get attention. Syphilis has no respect for his own body. Some people pierce or cut their bodies in **hidden places**—even on the sexual organs. One of my patients had some body part pierced for every trauma she went through in her life. What does this mean when she has to cut herself in response to receiving some shock or trauma? The healthy reaction is to mourn or cry—to grieve—and then, after some time, get the strength to overcome the trauma or repair her mistakes, because sometimes we cause our own traumas. This syphilitic patient who has experienced trauma gives herself another trauma by piercing her body. It is self-mutilation—causing pain and suffering to oneself, which is syphilitic. Many young people wear black. Some of it is fashion, but some are depressed and have no real joy in life. They say to their parents, "Why did you have me? You gave me such an awful life." This is the feeling of misery that runs throughout the syphilitic miasm.

While psora manifests as too little energy (weakness) and fear, syphilitic action is about destruction and perversion—**functioning in the wrong way**. Everyone has problems, and the normal reaction or functioning is to seek solutions from within or ask for help in solving the problems and move on. When syphilis has many problems, which he does not speak about, there is turmoil inside, and he gets depressed. He feels alone. He keeps dark secrets.

We may hear the syphilitic person say she cannot sleep well because of her depression or pains in the night. She is restless and tosses and turns. She lies on one side and then the other, rolling from side to side. She is sleepless, constantly moving, with thoughts that disturb her. Suicide may come to mind. She thinks, "If this is life, then I have to end it. I do not want to go on living." If she is less ill, Ms. Syphilis may suffer from depression and restless sleep, but without suicidal thoughts.

While psoric sleep is disturbed because of worry about tomorrow, syphilis may have **destructive thoughts**. He may think about hate or revenge. He may dream about his teeth rotting or falling out or about being bitten. He may dream about killing someone or doing something destructive. In the dream, he may kill the person chasing him, or something destructive may happen to his attacker—something may fall on her and kill her. A syphilitic mother may have a nightmare about killing her child. She is shocked that she can have this thought. It is the syphilitic part of her that speaks to her in the night.

What is normal human sexual behavior? Loving each other, liking to share bodies, wanting to be as close as possible. It gives happiness and joy, an extra dimension in life. At a certain age, the body, mind, and emotions are ripe to have a sexual life—enjoying sex, having children, and being happy with each other. However, these days, some may feel that this is an old-fashioned "fairy tale."

Homeopaths and psychiatrists often see destructive sexual expression—the most hidden part of human nature—in the illnesses of their patients. We sometimes treat people who have had or want to have sex with their own child. Incest or sexual abuse toward a child is syphilitic. Syphilitic people like to have sex in secret. Why? Some may believe that their sexual feelings are bad. Some may say they have difficulty connecting with people in what we would think is an acceptable or normal way. Some may have sex with animals. Some may prefer to have violent sex or have harmful sexual fantasies. Some syphilitic individuals buy or kidnap children to have sex with them and kill the child at the moment of orgasm because it gives extra stimulation. Some children's bodies have been used in this terrible way. This is the behavior of strongly perverted syphilitic people. These people are much more ill than those who only have the impulse to kill. Sadists and masochists are syphilitic. Syphilis causes perversion, doing things in the wrong way, keeping things inside instead of talking about them. Syphilis hides because "If I do not hide, people will see that I am bad and that I have bad wishes." **He hides, but he does not feel shame**. To rape, one must have the syphilitic miasm or the sycotic plus the syphilitic miasm. Sycosis may be very active sexually, but rape, which is a violent act, is syphilitic.

A predominantly psoric person with a bit of the syphilitic miasm might molest children—perhaps if he is too shy to share sex with an equal adult partner. But in this case the psoric offender will calm the child down after this awful behavior, give them treats, and try to be nice to them. He would never kill them.

I seldom ask patients about their sexual behavior directly because there are so many other symptoms evident from the rest of the body. But often a woman will be referred to me who asks for an appointment for her husband because of his sexual behavior. I then ask the husband to tell me about his own sexuality.

Repeated **alcohol** or other **drug problems** in the family history are indications of the syphilitic miasm. Syphilis may use alcohol to avoid his depressed feelings. He may become **violent after drinking** because alcohol stimulates his miasmatic tendency toward aggression. There are many problems with addictions in the syphilitic miasm—alcoholism and other drug addictions—people slowly destroying themselves, their families, and their lives. **Addictions** to excessive gambling, pain medications and sleeping pills, and abusive sexual practices are examples of syphilitic addiction. Having many **hidden secrets** in the family is syphilitic. A person often sends his or her syphilitic spouse to me to help them overcome the addiction, and if this person *wants* to stop something, a homeopathic remedy can strengthen his will.

Not every syphilitic person shows illness on these mental and emotional levels. Most have physical complaints.

General and Physical Symptoms and Modalities of the Syphilitic Miasm

Worse sunset to sunrise
Bone pain
Nighttime aggravation
Offensive discharges—fetid, rotten, stinking
Narrow parameters
Dulled senses
Hidden destruction
Destructive addictions
Sudden threat of death from disruption or dysfunction
Corrosion
Cracks
Grayish discharges
Bloody discharges
Eating away of tissue
Asymmetry
Deformity

The active hours of the syphilitic miasm are from 6:00 P.M. to 6:00 A.M.—sunset to sunrise. He is wide-awake in the evening, up late at night, and may sleep all day. His problems start at twilight. He may **dread** the night because his physical complaints worsen at night. Except for itching that burns, which is psoric, most nightly problems are syphilitic. Syphilis may be unable to sleep because of **bone pains or a feeling of coldness in the bones** or muscle cramps and spasms in the night. Seizures in the night are syphilitic.

Temperature is not specific for syphilis—she may be quite normal or a little cool. But if she is cold, it probably will not be the extreme cold of psora, although extremes of temperature in either direction bother syphilis. Her body has no flexibility, and she has **trouble maintaining the correct internal temperature**—she gets hot or cold too easily. She is worse if too warm or too cold. Her energy is mostly normal, but she often appears very **still, reserved, and controlled**. Her coloring may be gray. The sweating of syphilis is **stinking**. It is similar to the smell of cat or horse urine, and a homeopath may smell it in the consulting room. Syphilitic perspiration is very offensive (psoric sweat is sour). Natural **discharges** such as perspiration make psora feel better but tend to **aggravate** syphilis. While psora desires rich, fatty foods, syphilis desires smoked food (it has been smoked and is "deadened"). She also likes cold foods and drinks and may complain of a metallic or copper taste in her mouth.

Syphilis does not have the sensitivities of psora. Instead, his senses may be dulled. His sense of smell may be **dulled** or lost. Sometimes syphilis is cold, but he will not be able to say so because he is not in touch with his body.

Syphilis, both the disease and the miasm, causes the **breakdown of tissue** and the death of organs—in a **hidden** way. In the syphilitic miasm, there is silence and hiding, even in a **physical** way. For instance, his teeth may rot from underneath. Suddenly, he gets a pain or loses a tooth and finds that the whole root is rotten. He did not feel this as it was happening, but now it is there. This is how syphilis works with all the organs of the body. The danger that syphilis fears in his mind is mirrored in his body with **sudden, dangerous situations**. A neighbor who has never complained has a heart attack or stroke and dies suddenly. The disease had been going on, he did not complain, and suddenly his life is finished. With little notice, syphilis begins feeling unwell, goes to the doctor, is sent to the hospital for tests that uncover advanced disease, and three weeks later she is dead from cancer. This is not psora; this is syphilis. Syphilitic people burn out very soon.

Syphilis is **perversion, disruption, or dysfunction**. In syphilis there is a tendency to sudden blockage of the internal organs. Disruption of the urinary or bowel function is syphilitic. Alzheimer's disease (AD) is a syphilitic disease because it **destroys** the brain function. (It can come from suppression due to blood pressure medicine or sleeping pills.) We may recognize syphilis in multiple sclerosis (MS), because the nerves are being destroyed. MS can kill someone who is quite young, another syphilitic indication. The hidden grief of syphilis may cause this kind of nerve damage. He becomes paralyzed on the physical level. We need to discover and remove these dangerous possibilities in our syphilitic patients. But does this mean that we should treat all of our AD and MS patients with syphilitic remedies? No. It depends on how the patient presents. It depends on the total symptom picture.

Remember that we are not treating the disease itself. We can classify diseases as their symptoms relate to certain miasms, but we must always give a remedy that addresses the patient's state if we are to remove the symptoms of the disease.

The syphilitic lung infection is **destructive**, like the lung inflammations of years ago, when the doctor sat by the bed watching over the patient because many patients died of these lung infections. Syphilitic asthma has grayish mucus that is difficult to expectorate, with strong spasms during the night.

Discharges in syphilitic illnesses are mostly **grayish and bloody** or yellow with red color, because syphilis breaks down the organism. The syphilitic miasm shows bloody, broken things. A hemangioma is syphilitic. Bleeding hemorrhoids are syphilitic. Any easy tendency to bleed is mostly syphilitic, and sometimes the blood is dark.

When syphilis has an ear infection, she does not mention it, and then suddenly there is pain and an infection with a stinking smell that is almost too offensive to believe. (The psoric ear infection does not stink.) The syphilitic ear infection comes on at twilight and builds up during the night. The discharge is grayish, with some blood. The infection is **corrosive**, going inside. The eardrum breaks. These are ear infections that can destroy the ear. In a psoric case, there is time to study. In a syphilitic case, there is little time, and the infection may be dangerous. About these infections, allopaths say, "You are a fool to use homeopathy. You might destroy the ear." On the contrary, if we give the correct syphilitic remedy, there will be no destruction and the patient will not have problems with the ear anymore. Recurrent syphilitic ear infections can cause deafness. Syphilis may cause **distortion** of vision, and syphilitic eye infections may destroy the inner eye. Strep throat is syphilitic when the fever occurs at night and there are holes in the tonsils or there is a lot of **gray pus** mixed with blood.

Within the syphilitic miasm, there may be **deep canker** sores on the lips and gums. Psoric patients may complain of little sores or ulcers in or on the mouth that are painful, red, and burning, but a syphilitic canker sore creates a **deep hole** and stinks. The tissue in the mouth is **rotting** away. The sores are not red but gray and heal very slowly. These sores can heal only when the syphilitic miasm is treated.

Imagine that an allopath prescribes an allopathic drug for the patient with a canker sore. If the patient is syphilitic and the canker sore goes away because of a suppressive medication, the sore may show up in another area. It also is likely that the newly affected area will be **hidden**, perhaps deeper inside. Perhaps the patient's ancestors have had stomach problems. After the patient's canker sores are gone, he may go back to the doctor for stomach problems because the tendency is in his family. The problems go to the patient's weakness or to the level of illness within the family history.

In the disease of syphilis, there is the "true" ulcer. Miasmatically, syphilitic ulcers become holes that eat away the skin. When a hole in the skin is a dirty gray color, with some blood, it is a sign of the syphilitic miasm. Aphthae that look like gray holes in the mouth are syphilitic. **Colitis ulcerosa** is syphilitic.

Some people get a **syphilitic fistula** that eats down into the tissue. These may be very deep. Once I saw a patient with a fistula in the buttock. The nurse told me she could put her whole hand down into it. Some fistulas that are treated allopathically, by cleaning and draining, may eventually clear, but the problem will go deeper. To what level? Maybe to an ulcer in the stomach, which is harder to cure. Stomach ulcers are mostly syphilitic. Why does the organism make the problem go deeper? The imbalance or disruption in the organism that created the need for the fistula to form did so as a last resort, so to speak. Clearing the fistula does not clear the underlying imbalance that remains in need of expression.

The body shows its troubles only through symptoms, and when these symptoms are treated on a superficial level and thus suppressed, the vital force must deal with the problem somewhere else, in some other way.

Perhaps the fistula was the best solution found by the vital force; but now, after suppressing this outlet, the organism must find another solution. So far, I have seen a complete level of cure occur only with homeopathy.

Cirrhosis of the liver exhibits syphilitic traits. Initially, the tissue swells, then hardens, and then is destroyed. Diabetes is partly syphilitic because it involves destruction of the cells, but it is a combination of all the miasms.

A heart attack in which the **veins rupture** is syphilitic. Irregular heartbeat is syphilitic because it is a dysfunction of the heart. The heart problems of syphilis may build silently until there is an **unexpected breakdown**. High blood pressure is mostly sycotic, but it has elements of the psoric, syphilitic, and sycotic miasms.

A syphilitic eruption occurs under the skin and eats into the body. Syphilitic warts occur under the skin, **growing inward**—plantar warts; they are hiding. Only a little point of the wart is seen on the surface; the rest is under the skin. These occur in the history of syphilitic patients. Usually, the warts are removed in some way—burned off, cut out, or chemically frozen. Crusts and scabs in syphilis tend to be thick and heavy.

Vitiligo is syphilitic. Healthy skin is mostly uniform in color all over the body, but in vitiligo there are white-colored spots on the skin, where small or large portions of the pigment have been destroyed. In the allopathic understanding, vitiligo is considered an autoimmune disorder that is genetically inherited. All autoimmune diseases are syphilitic, because they are conditions where a person's immune system attacks itself and/or destroys the body's own cells, tissue or organs. This destruction is sign of the syphilitic miasm. In the case of vitiligo, the immune system attacks and damages or destroys melanocytes, which are responsible for producing melanin. When there is syphilis in the family history, it may express itself in vitiligo. When we look at the range of possible syphilitic problems, vitiligo is less serious than kidney failure, diabetes, or suicidal tendencies. Nevertheless, it is syphilitic.

Cracks in the skin are syphilitic and may be very painful. The skin breaks and bleeds. Most bleeding belongs to syphilis. There may be cracks in the corners of the mouth, in the nose, and between the toes. These may be deep, bleeding cracks. There also may be splits in the nails. A psoric person may scratch his skin until it burns, but a syphilitic person may scratch until it bleeds.

Hair loss can be syphilitic. How does a syphilitic person lose her hair? Perhaps after an illness or a trauma that is "cured" with allopathic drugs. Or she may pull it out. Or she may lose it after childbirth. Sometimes there is a partial loss of hair, which syphilis may try to hide. It is a secret. She may ask the homeopath for a hair loss remedy.

The syphilitic face may be **asymmetrical**. There may be one brown and one blue eye. Thin lips like a stripe are syphilitic. The nose may be too small (too little bone), because syphilis destroys bone tissue or **impedes** the organism's ability to build the correct tissue. A pointed chin that is very severe and sharp is syphilitic, as is a jaw that is too severly pointed, missing the square shape.

Syphilis causes degenerative muscle problems such as muscular dystrophy. There may be contractions and indurations as in Dupuytren's disease.

About 40 years ago, many women (of all miasms) who were sleepless during pregnancy were prescribed Thalidomide, which was withdrawn from general use after it was found to cause severe birth defects. Syphilitic mothers-to-be who took this drug (perhaps they could not sleep due to violent dreams or toothaches or other bone pains) sometimes had children with a syphilitic defect. Psoric mothers who took this drug might have babies who would develop more weakness. Miasmatically, the results of suppression are very logical.

Tranquilizers and antidepressants also may cause suppression. Vaccinations affect some children very badly, although other children are able to handle them with no serious reaction. If all children experienced problems after vaccination, it would be easier to prove that the practice of vaccination is harmful, and perhaps routine vaccination would cease. The same is true for alcohol or tobacco smoke. If everyone was badly affected by the same substance, most would not use it. But how badly we are affected depends on our vulnerability.

There is a joke about a newspaper reporter who interviewed an 80-year-old man. The reporter asked the old man what he did to stay in such good shape. "I exercise every day, I eat natural food, I don't smoke, and I don't drink, and that is why I have lived this long." As the reporter was writing this down, he heard a loud cough in the background. So he asked the old man, "Is that your wife?" The old man answered, "No, that is my father. He's a smoker." A man who has taken care of himself all his life has reason to be in good condition at 80 years old, especially if he is psoric. To live to be 98 as a smoker shows that his father was not so susceptible to tobacco smoke. Miasmatically, alcohol is most destructive to syphilitic people. They start drinking because they feel better when they drink, but it harms them.

There are many bone problems in syphilis, including **bone pain and bone deformation**. There may be **bone caries, cysts in the bones, osteoporosis, cancer in the bones**, and so on. The patient may be missing a rib bone, a finger bone, or other bone. The pain felt in the bones may be worse at night. There may be knock-knees, bowlegs, or bones that break easily. A patient of mine broke her ankle by simply stepping down from the curb onto the street. This occurred after the death of a child. There was silent grief with indifference to everything—even to her other children. She also lost her hair.

Syphilis holds **emotions inside, unexpressed**, and these hidden and suppressed emotional stresses may build up to break the bones. Although this is not allopathic understanding, homeopaths know that illness begins on the energetic level. By the time illness expresses itself on the physical level, as in the breaking of a bone by a simple step, the true illness has been there for some time. We can set the bone and allow the body to repair the break, but the illness goes on. Unless we can cure the inner disturbance, the potential for another break is great. If we do not understand that such a miasmatic illness in our patients is syphilitic, we might decide that this bone break is due to a lack of calcium or poor calcium uptake. The patient's allopath may prescribe added calcium or increased hormone, or her homeopath might prescribe a psoric remedy. If the patient is syphilitic, not only will her illness go on without relief, but if treated with a psoric remedy, the illness of her syphilitic state may be pushed to produce even more serious syphilitic symptoms.

Teeth can tell us much about a patient's miasm; however, dental work may have hidden the patient's formerly uncompensated dental features/problems. We should ask our patients about dental work, tendency to tooth decay, and orthodontic work. We sometimes see patients with a large space between the front teeth or big **spaces** between the other teeth. This is syphilitic. Syphilitic teeth are **serrated**, and the teeth may crack or crumble. Teeth that are not in the correct position or are at different angles, requiring orthodontic work, are syphilitic, as is a jaw that is too narrow. In syphilis, cavities may occur in hidden places, decaying from the inside or at the root of the tooth rather than on the surface. Teeth that become loose in the gums may be a syphilitic symptom because it indicates a dysfunctional process: The gums and teeth aren't behaving properly.

The syphilitic miasm can include **missing teeth** or teeth that erupt in an unusual order. The shapes of the gums and teeth can show miasmatic influence. In syphilis, the palate is often narrower and more elongated. An allopath may think these people need their mouths extended or widened to make room for the teeth or to correct the bite. Syphilitic patients give a lot of money to their dentists. They have more dental work than the other miasms.

Syphilitic tongues are cracked, sometimes giving the impression that someone has tried to chop up the tongue. One of my patients told me, "People are afraid of seeing my tongue because it is like chopped meat." There was the impression that her tongue needed repair because the cracks were so deep and red.

The Syphilitic Miasm in Infants and Children

When Baby Syphilis is born, he may have a **tiny head, be old looking, have a gray face, and lack one toe**—not a big problem since he can put on socks and shoes and no one will notice. His little ear may be **slightly deformed**; some distortion often occurs in syphilitic children. Baby Syphilis **cries** as soon as he is born. Every child cries: Baby Psora needs to be held; Baby Sycosis needs to be bounced, but little Baby Syphilis **cannot be consoled.** There is an emotional distance. It is as if he does not feel that he is loved. He cannot be calmed down. He cries all night. **Crying in the night** is one of the most prominent symptoms in syphilitic children. At some point he may stop crying because he gives up, feeling that it is hopeless. He does not seem to need his mother. He internalizes his needs. He does not start to laugh at six or seven weeks of age. He perspires, and it is a **stinking smell.** Little snuffles start, and there is **pus that is grayish**—pus in the eyes and pus on the fingernails. Mother takes Baby Syphilis to the doctor, who says "Pus, infection, inflammation, bacteria: He needs antibiotics." A child's vitality is often suppressed with immunizations, and symptoms are suppressed with antibiotics. What happens with Baby Syphilis after the antibiotics? His nose clears, the infection is gone, and now he is "only" sleepless. At four or five years of age, he no longer has snuffles with gray pus, but something more serious, more dangerous, more life threatening—perhaps a serious kidney block.

Child Syphilis is not like his psoric cousin who likes to make contact with everyone. Child Syphilis sits **alone**, plays alone, and is a depressed child. It is strange and awful to see his sad eyes and his inability to play with others. Because of anger or frustration, he may **bang his head** against the wall. When he does make contact with someone, it is usually by **fighting**. He breaks things and cannot express himself through his feelings, only through actions. When these syphilitic children become overactive and are given a drug to control their activity, the restlessness may stop, but the problem then goes to the mind. They may become capable of crime. Even syphilitic children as young as three or four years old may exhibit threatening behavior, because their syphilitic miasm has been suppressed and their **illness has gone deeper** into the mind.

I have been "shot" at many times in my consulting room. A little boy comes in with his mother and pretends to shoot me with his finger or a toy gun. He may have a big smile and show me his "big gun." This may be a fearful psoric child who feels better because he has a toy gun and can show strength. A syphilitic child comes in shooting with that same pointed finger or toy gun, but with hate on his face because he has to go to a homeopath with his mother, or he may stand behind his mother, hiding and glaring. His eyes are cold. I look at him and feel as if I am watching a violent movie. It is chilling to see coldness and hate in the eyes of a child. Our first contact and observation can tell us a lot.

When asked about her child, the mother of a syphilitic child may say that her son chokes the dog or pulls the legs off of insects. She may say, "He is fond of his little sister, but I cannot leave him alone with her because he puts his hands around her neck." Syphilitic children may break things and destroy their toys, have **outbursts of anger**, be physically **aggressive**, and irritate others constantly. They may make **dark or violent drawings** with guns and knives. A young patient of one of my colleagues drew a picture for her of a sea, sand dunes, and a sky with very dark clouds. The plants were brown. The picture looked threatening. Some time after giving the child his syphilitic remedy, his improvement was reflected in the peaceful nature of his next drawing.

A baby who is born with **septicemia** or with convulsive hands and feet or who continuously vomits all his food and cries all night is syphilitic. A child who has trouble breathing in the night is syphilitic. The teeth of syphilitic babies may come through in an unusual order, and new ones may come in before the old ones fall out. They may be **born with teeth**, which is not normal development.

Children with growing pains or who wake up with pain in the tibia are syphilitic. They can walk, jump, and play during the day, but at night they wake up screaming.

Birth defects can occur in syphilitic babies. They may be missing a toe, have a cleft palate, have only one kidney, or have an organ out of place, such as the heart on the wrong side. Syphilitic babies can show **strange mistakes** in the body: Internal tubes may be twisted, the foot may be twisted and turned out, one leg may be a little shorter, the spine may be deformed, a vertebra may be missing, or there may be too few or too many fingers and toes. A baby born with the umbilical cord around the neck may be syphilitic. When the family has a strong syphilitic miasm, the miasm may show itself at the moment of birth.

As the child grows, the psoric child may have a history of being tired or having an itch. After suppression of any of her symptoms, the result may be more tiredness, more itch, more disturbances. If the child is syphilitic, with a family history of Crohn's disease or if a family member has committed **suicide**, the future for this syphilitic baby is potentially more serious. Children can inherit the tendency toward the same disease as their ancestors. Sometimes a child will try to commit suicide. The youngest patient in our practice who attempted suicide was five years old; he tried to hang himself on the door. He had a prior history of mild illnesses, but there also had been suicide in his family.

Suppose a baby or young child has the active syphilitic miasm, and she inherits a family background of kidney or intestinal problems. If she begins to have diarrhea or a kidney infection and her symptoms are suppressed with seemingly innocent allopathic medicines, her illness, which may have looked like an innocent childhood illness, can result in colitis or kidney failure. Even cancer may occur in such a child of only two or three years of age. There is a lot of cancer in children because they are not being treated in a way that builds up their energy. Instead, their energy is being blocked or cut off.

Miasms in Pregnancy

We can learn to recognize how miasmatic expressions manifest in our pregnant patients. Women experience many changes during pregnancy. A woman may feel a change in her own state during pregnancy, which is the effect of carrying a child who is of a different miasmatic makeup than her own. For example, if a primarily psoric woman marries a man with a syphilitic miasm, their baby may be psoric if the mother is strong, but syphilitic if the father is stronger, or a combination of both. Most of the time, both states go into the "pot." If a psoric mother is pregnant with a syphilitic baby, she may show the state of the baby. She may have syphilitic symptoms during her pregnancy. If the mother is syphilitic, her state will not be changed by carrying a psoric baby. The best thing for unborn children is to treat the mother while she is pregnant. The child will be born with better health. If the mother changes from one state to another during her pregnancy, she usually goes back to her original state after the baby is born.

Bleeding during pregnancy and the tendency to abort are mostly syphilitic. The blood may be dark, almost black. Some syphilitic women cannot carry their babies to full term. If a woman's ligaments and bones cannot hold a baby, she must stay in a wheelchair or in bed from about six weeks on. This is very syphilitic. Having more than two fetuses is syphilitic.

When a syphilitic person and a psoric person have children, there will be a mixture of miasms in their children. One child might be more syphilitic and less psoric; another might be more psoric and less syphilitic. If a syphilitic person marries another syphilitic person, the syphilitic miasm will be even stronger in their children. The only way to decrease the syphilitic miasm is for psora to marry only psora or to treat everyone homeopathically.

Syphilitic Remedies

To learn the syphilitic remedies, start with *Kent's Repertory*. **GENERALITIES; SYPHILIS** (48): **Ars-i.**, **Aur.**, **Aur-m.**, **Aur-m-n.**, **Kali-i.**, **Kali-s.**, **Merc.**, **Merc-c.**, **Merc-i-f.**, **Merc-i-r.**, **Nit-ac.**, **Phyt.**, **Sil.**, **Still.**, **Syph.**, *ars.*, *ars-s-f.*, *asaf.*, *calc-i.*, *calc-s.*, *carb-an.*, *cinnb.*, *con.*, *fl-ac.*, *hep.*, *iod.*, *kali-ar.*, *kali-bi.*, *kali-chl.*, *lach.*, *led.*, *mez.*, *ph-ac.*, *phos.*, *sars.*, *staph.*, *sul-i.*, *sulph.*, *thuj.*, arg., bad., benz-ac., carb-v., clem., cor-r., crot-h., guai., petr.

In *Kent's Repertory*, even the nine remedies in plain type in the "Syphilis" rubric are trustworthy. In the new repertories, we can rely on those in bold type, and most in Italics are reliable. Another way to learn is to look at the proving symptoms of the remedies and compare those symptoms with those of the miasm. Decide to which miasms each of the symptoms belongs. No remedy is totally psoric, sycotic, or syphilitic. All have symptoms of each of the miasms, but most are stronger in one or another.

Syphilinum is the nosode of the syphilitic miasm. It has many of the symptoms of the syphilitic miasm, of course, but it is not the only remedy with which to treat this miasm profoundly. Some other remedies that are very strong in syphilitic symptoms are *Aurum metallicum, Mercurius vivus, Mercurius corrosivus,* and *Nitricum acidum.* Some symptoms of *Syphilinum* are:

- Distrust of other people and of oneself
- Fear of contamination, delusion one is dirty, always washing one's hands
- Fear of paralysis (mental or physical)
- Desire for alcohol. Alcoholism (especially if it is in the family history)
- Aversion to consolation
- Dullness, in children
- Difficulty doing calculations
- Nightly aggravation, worse sunset to sunrise
- Prostration and debility in the morning
- Bone pains
- Deformations of the body
- Ulceration with foul discharges

Syphilis Case 1: Baby Girl With Reflux and Thrush

Video Presentation and Case Description

The following discussion was captured as it occurred during a video presentation and case description by Henny Heudens. Student questions and comments appear in brackets in italics.

I first saw this little girl when she was two-and-a-half months old. She is trying to stand in her daddy's lap, and the mother sits next to them. The consultation lasted for more than one hour. Almost the whole time, she was standing against her father. I thought this was very early for her to stand, but she seemed fine in that position. The baby watches her mother all the time and watches me. I am behind the camera, and she follows me with her eyes, as she does again when the phone rings. Before we talk with them, what do you think is strange, rare, and peculiar (SRP)? [*She is being held by the dad rather than the mother.*] Is this what you normally expect in a consultation? How is this father? Sympathetic and proud. What impression do you have when you see the family? The child looks like the father. The baby's father is very sweet and loving. In my entire professional life, I've never (that I can remember) seen a father who was so sweet with his little child. The father behaves as a sweet mother would. He protects the child. The mother phoned and asked us to see her baby because her friend, a homeopath, told her to come to us.

What is the baby's problem? Reflux. She vomits all her food. Her problem is not only vomiting but thrush in the mouth and in the esophagus. The thrush began in her mouth, but after allopathic drugs, it went to the esophagus. The mother's friend told her not to treat the child allopathically anymore because the problem would go deeper. She suggested that the mother try herbs and take the child to a homeopath. There is a rubric in *Kent's Repertory* **MOUTH; APHTHAE; *children, in,*** but we never start a case with such a rubric. We have wonderful remedies for thrush: *Borax*, for example. But if this is not a *Borax* child, the problem will be suppressed, and the fungus will go deeper. We have to hear the case.

Why did the baby get this fungus right after birth? My attention goes to the mother. The mother took a fertility drug to get pregnant, and before that she took birth control pills not to be pregnant. The mother got a vaginal fungus during pregnancy in the fifth or sixth month. It was treated with antibiotics and antifungal medication. The fungus was suppressed. She had a difficult delivery—after 30 hours of labor the os would not open. The mother was very tired, and they used forceps. When using the forceps, there was a big tear (perineum and neck of uterus), and immediately they gave her antibiotics after birth due to the possibility of infection. The baby was unconscious at birth and had an Apgar score of 5. She was blue, initially not breathing. But within five minutes she recovered and had a score of 10. The mother breastfed the baby while on antibiotics (her doctors told her it would be safe), and the baby developed a fungus. The mother is currently breastfeeding the baby, and the baby weeps and vomits and has thrush. This baby has had a bad start.

Do you see how cramped the father looks—the postural position he is willing to take to make the baby comfortable? How is she at two-and-a-half months of age? Are there any pediatricians here? [*I think she looks good. Some babies don't move at all at this age.*] Is she average, better than average? [*Better than average.*] I think so; she is even precocious for her age, more advanced than usual. She is doing well for her age. She has very nice skin and is tiny and delicate. She is serious, not smiling at all, and is very alert. In the evening she is restless from about 8:00 P.M. to 9:00 P.M., and the father says she needs her pacifier. She cries a little, and they give it to her. He says she always has cold hands and feet. When I ask what she does not like to do, he says she does not like being dressed or bathed because she is awfully cold. She does not like sleeping on her abdomen; she always lies on her back. She has hiccups a lot, mostly after laughing. In the beginning, her stool occurred every day, but now she has only one in three days and has a lot of flatus. She loves a lot of contact. Do we think this is true? [*Definitely.*] In her sleep, she starts from the least noise. She shrieks sometimes and throws her hands high, and then she wakes. She falls asleep, starts with a quick movement, and then falls asleep again. Sometimes she weeps in her sleep. Sometimes she laughs in her sleep. When I ask what she definitely does not like, the father says that when she makes stool she starts to cry. They have to change her quickly. She loves to be with her parents, and she feels fine when they are near.

One week after birth, the fungus started on the baby's lips, then on her tongue, then (after drug treatment) in the esophagus. She was treated with Nystatin. With Nystatin she can eat, but she vomits a lot. The vomiting is very sour and thick like curdled milk or yogurt, and it stinks. The father says she is a beautiful child and very sweet and only weeps when she needs to. The mother says she did not want to give Nystatin because the baby did not like it, but after some time the child liked to take it. The father worries about the baby taking Nystatin. He says that maybe she will become dependent on it. He says she moves some but is really quite calm. The mother says, "She has caught a cold because it was freezing this winter, and our house is not well insulated." She caught a cold because she slept in a cold room. They felt they had to put her in the living room, which was warmer—then the cold went away. They had to cover her a lot because she did not like the cold. She coughed, and her nose was blocked. The father said he is amazed that she feels so cold. Since she had an Apgar score of 5 and she recovered so quickly, he thought she had energy. He asks, "Why are her hands and feet so cold?"

The mother says that perhaps they have forgotten something. "Ah yes," the father said, "Her little feet at birth were a little twisted. The doctors said not to worry, that the foot had been in the wrong direction in the uterus." The father mentions it anyway. The right foot is not quite right; it turns outward. Also, the children's specialist said that the child might be backward because of the birth and instructed the parents to bring the child in every three months for evaluation. They hope to be able to determine her ability by age six or seven years. This is an awful message to receive as a parent. Imagine how this affects them? The baby is too young to speak, so we can only observe. She seems to be a sweet baby. It is an easy case; beginners can give the solution, but I'd like for us to do this in a miasmatic way.

Syphilis Case 1—Analysis

We often see children with a similar history, and many of them have had antibiotics for illnesses several times by the time they are three months old. What are the strange symptoms—what is characteristic for this baby, and what else do we have to know? [*Her miasm*]. Let's discuss.

The family history is nothing special. The father had nothing unusual. The mother had problems getting pregnant. What else? The doctor said the baby was in a strange position in the uterus. What child is in a strange position in a soft, comfortable uterus? Not all babies are born with their foot twisted. This is very syphilitic. If you did not know this, you would definitely prescribe a psoric remedy. But we have this little syphilitic symptom. Is she only syphilitic? [*No, she is also psoric: sour smell, coldness, etc.*] It would be nice if we could find a remedy that covered both. What symptoms are psoric? [*The baby is cold.*] Yes. A baby should be warm, or else it is SRP. When an old woman is very hot, this is a symptom, but a baby should normally be warm.

This baby's symptoms are:

- Syphilitic background
- Coldness

- Hiccups from laughing
- Precocious
- Starts in her sleep

Can you imagine a baby who does this? Why? She is easily startled and has a strong reaction; this means that her neurological area is weak. [*Also, she cries after stool.*] The father says that she does not like to be dressed, but after stool she cries because she needs a clean diaper. It means that she is **fastidious**. Is it normal for a baby to cry when it makes stool? No; they are used to this. She only makes stool once every three or four days. For a breastfed child, this is not so peculiar. However, crying after making stool to warn the parents is unusual. She does not like the diaper full of stool; she is fastidious. [*How do you know it's not pain?*] If there is pain, babies usually cry during stool or when their bottom is hurt and made red by the stool.

The patient likes to be with her father (more than with her mother), and the father wants to be with the child. How does the father hold the baby? He has large hands and holds her under her bottom, and she likes it. I have the feeling he feels how delicate she is and wants to protect her. Maybe she likes the pressure of his big hands, and maybe she likes the security. We need a cold remedy, a precocious remedy, where the picture includes cold hands and feet. We need a remedy that likes to be very neat and clean and that cries after stool. What rubric can we use for this? [*Conscientious about trifles.*] A diaper with stool is a trifle for the average baby, and for this baby this trifle is important. This baby is cold and weak and needs the strength of the father's big hands. Our correct remedy has all these symptoms. From the Materia Medica, some symptoms for this case are:

- Shrieks during sleep, throws hands high
- Psora + syphilis
- Sleeps on back
- Delicate
- Cold hands and feet (SRP for a baby)
- Fastidious
- Conscientious about trifles/disgust—hates mess in diapers
- Serious
- Quiet
- Desires company

- Vomiting thick, sour, and stinking
- Laughing during sleep
- Hiccups after laughing
- Medicines—abuse of drugs
- Pain in mother at birth

Which of the following is the most important?
- Baby feels cold (SRP for a baby).
- She is fastidious (SRP for a baby).
- She shrieks, starts, and laughs in her sleep. This is due to immaturity of the nervous system of the baby.

Rubrics that can be used are:
- EXTREMITIES; JERKING; *sleep; agg.; during*
- STOMACH; VOMITING; *milk; curdled*
- MIND; LAUGHING; *general; sleep; during*
- MIND; ANXIETY; *trifles, about*
- GENERALITIES; COLD; *becoming; agg*
- EXTREMITIES; COLDNESS; *general; icy; lower limbs; feet*
- MOUTH; APHTHAE

And we have both the syphilitic and psoric miasm.

Some possible remedies are [*student suggestions*]:
- *Silica*
- *Lycopodium*
- *Arsenicum*
- *Thuja*
- *Calcarea phosphorica*

How would a *Thuja* baby be? She would be worse at night. *Thuja* is sensitive to wet, but this weather was very dry and cold. Also, *Thuja* is strongly sycotic (as is *Medorrhinum*), and we are looking for a remedy with psora and syphilis. We would need strong sycotic symptoms to prescribe *Thuja.*

How is *Calcarea phosphorica*? Dissatisfied, peevish. This baby is not like that. With *Arsenicum,* there is nighttime aggravation and coldness, but this baby is not restless and not anxious at all. She is very secure.

Lycopodium has flatulence and some vomiting. With *Lycopodium*, flatus must be very strong. But *Lycopodium* likes things in the mouth, and she does not like to suck on her finger, only on the pacifier at night when she is tired. She gets tired in the evening. Also, *Lycopodium* babies weep. They are not very satisfied or peaceful, and she is both.

Silica remains, and this is a typical *Silica* baby. She has delicacy, sour nature, seriousness, not moving a lot, shrieks during sleep, conscientious about trifles, and laughs during sleep. *Silica* is listed as a strongly psoric and syphilitic remedy.

Does she look like a *Silica* baby? Yes, very delicate. Think about the Materia Medica. How does *Silica* behave? When one is focused on trifles, as *Silica* is, one is serious. When *Silica* does things, it is in a very serious way. In my experience, there is a lot of fungus in *Silica*. Think about their nails. Their nails are cracked and have fungus. Never prescribe *Silica* only for fungus, but it is nice to know this, just as it is nice to know that *Lycopodium* usually has problems in the stomach. Silica babies may have deformed bones. The head feels different, and you can feel the openings and bones. The skin is delicate and tight on the bones. There is the impression that there is no meat. The head looks big because they are so tiny elsewhere. They are often constipated, and this baby has one stool in three days. There is also weakness throughout.

Regarding thrush in the mouth, in *Kent's Repertory* under **MOUTH; APHTHAE; *children, in,*** *Silica* is not listed (although it is listed under **MOUTH, APHTHAE**). When you start looking for symptoms in an allopathic, diagnostic way, you will be misled.

I gave two doses of *Silica* 200C—one immediately and the other to take home. We stopped the Nystatin. What will be the result after the *Silica*? [*The thrush will come back.*] The mother cannot see the thrush in the esophagus, but after the remedy, we know that it will come into the mouth; babies with a lot of pain from aphthae complain. If she does not drink, she will dehydrate. If the thrush comes back and the baby cannot bear it, then the parents will do something else to get rid of it. I know it has to come back. Better to give them a spare dose and tell them that I expect the thrush to come back. They don't have to do anything unless the child cannot bear it. When she cannot bear it, they have to contact me, and they definitely have to phone me five days after the remedy. This is for reassurance only. I want the parents to know they are not being sent away without help.

Syphilis Case 1—Followups

The mother phones on Friday and says, "She does not jerk or laugh anymore in her sleep. She has a lot of fungus in her mouth. What should I do?" The baby is drinking, and the vomiting is less. Would you repeat the remedy? [*No.*] You have to listen to everything the parents say. Where has the remedy worked? Her nervous system is stronger in only four days. She sleeps better, without jerking. There is a return of the old thrush in the mouth, but the baby drinks. I tell the mother not to do anything and to call me again on Monday. When the mother calls on Monday, the thrush is better. The baby sleeps well and eats well. I expect it will disappear. I tell her to phone me again later.

The mother called three weeks after the remedy. Everything is finished. The thrush is gone, the child is fine, and she makes stool every day. She is improving. The father calls for an appointment for his problems. That is when I hear how amazing it was that the child changed temperature! Two weeks after the remedy, a lot of sweat came out of her feet. Her feet were wet, then dried up, and her feet and hands became warm. Now the vitality of the child is good because she is healthy. He said, "You can't imagine how stinking the sweat was that came out of the baby's feet. It was awful!" The mother said, "The nice thing after the remedy was that two weeks afterward, I had to cut her nails for the first time." The mother had never told me that the baby's nails had never grown. The remedy stimulated growth.

The child is now about 15 months old and has not been ill since her first dose of the remedy. She is fine and has not been vaccinated. We had a telephone call about that. I told the mother not to have the child vaccinated because she could have a big aggravation afterward. Is it so remarkable that the remedy took away the fungus? We did not give her *Borax*, or a strongly syphilitic remedy such as *Mercury*, but *Silica.*

What would have happened if we had suppressed her? If the thrush went down quickly without other improvement, the thrush might have gone to the lungs or the intestines. The vital force chooses where the remedy must work. The jerking was more important than the thrush, and we must remember that vaccinations are very difficult for babies who have this type of jerking.

I prefer the remedy to be taken when a patient can rest afterward. This family was going to travel a long way, and the baby appeared tired. I told them to give it to her at home. Normally, I would have given it to the mother if she were nursing, but this baby's remedy suited the father more than the mother. To administer to children, I tell the parents to crush the pills to powder and put this powder inside the lip of the child. This child is fine, and one year has passed since the remedy.

I do not know how she will develop. She went back to the hospital for tests. Specialists are much higher in the hierarchy than homeopaths. But it will not harm her to be looked at. If they had recommended a spinal tap or another procedure, I would have told the parents to think about it. [*Would you have given something when the baby was unconscious at birth?*] If I were present at the birth, I would have definitely given a remedy. Homeopaths are not often present. Frequently I am called when there is a problem. I speak to the mother or, if not possible, to the father, and I can often can prescribe over the phone in these cases when the picture is clear. The best way to treat a baby is to treat the parents before conception. If you treat the mother, even during pregnancy, the baby will be much better.

Syphilis Case 2: Six-Year-Old Boy With Pervasive Developmental Delay

Live Case Presentation

This live case, taken by Henny Heudens (HH) before seminar students, is presented in its entirety as an initial consult, with case analysis and followup. Students' questions and comments appear in italics within brackets. Nonitalicized words in parentheses were added by the transcriber to clarify meaning. Some other words are in italics for emphasis. "PH" indicates "presenting homeopath."

Family History

Father's side:

- Grandmother has history of skin cancer.
- Grandfather is 84, with a history of allergies, stomach ulcer, and Rosacea.
- Both great-grandparents died of cancer.
- Alcoholism.

Mother's side:

- Alcoholism
- Emphysema
- Skin cancer
- Breast cancer

HH—Hello, Kevin. It's nice that you visit us. (He screams and tries to leave. He screams again. His mother says that he likes to be outside. He picks up a paper from the table.)

HH—Hi, Kevin. We heard a little history. (He climbs up on stage now.) Nice that you are with us.

HH (to his mother)—What do you find to be the biggest problem in him?

Mother—He has no reasoning. You can't just run out in the street. He does not seem to get that. There is no fear. He's not afraid of anything. He'll climb to the top of anything.

HH—No fear of even water, for example, or sounds?

Mother—Just recently, he does not want his hair washed. He likes water but does not like to go swimming in the pool. He likes to pour it from one cup to another. He likes to stand at the sink, play in the water, and wash dishes.

HH—He has brothers and sisters?

Mother—He is the fourth. He is right there with them; he has to be in that room with them.

HH—How does he react then?

Mother—He stands at the door and screams. If he does not get anything, he screams.

HH—Is there anything that makes him happy?

Mother—If he's getting his way, he's real happy. He likes to be outside all the time. He wanders around, looks at things, touches everything, rides his tricycle, pushes things around. (He touches and picks up everything.) He has no interest in animals.

HH—What kind of toys does he like?

Mother—Cars, things with wheels. He flips books in his face. Wants a book all the time.

HH—When he is doing this, what do you think he is doing? Smelling the books?

Mother—He's brushing his face, or he likes the feel of the air.

HH—When he plays with cars, how does he play?

Mother—He pushes them around, makes a sound. He likes to roll them down the steps and stuff.

HH—He has no fear of people?

Mother—No. We thought he couldn't hear, and we had his hearing checked. (It is all right.) He runs for the commercials, likes to watch the credits scroll at the ends of movies.

HH—How can you touch him? (He smiles for the camera.)

Mother—He's lovable, likes to be held. He likes attention. He's laughing with the camera on him. When we do the blessing at dinner, he thinks that it's for him.

HH—When he is screaming, how can you calm him down?

Mother—Screaming at him helps. If I put him in the bathtub, he's instantly happy. In restaurants and shops, he wants to do his own thing, and when he can't he's not happy.

HH—He likes the bathtub. What temperature?

Mother—He'll sit in it if it's cold or warm. He likes the water on and does not like for me to turn it off.

HH—How is he sleeping?

Mother—When he sleeps, he sleeps very well. Getting him there is the problem. He likes to stay up late and sleep late.

HH—Do you have to put him down physically?

Mother—He screams and then throws up. He gets so upset, he throws up. Then we let him get up.

HH—What does he throw up?

Mother—Whatever he's had to eat—liquid, water, tea. He sucks on his shirt all the time. (He starts flipping the book on his face.) He does this especially when he's irritable or tired.

HH—Does he recognize pictures?

Mother—No. He does not recognize things.

HH—Once he's asleep, does he sleep all night long without waking or making sounds?

Mother—Yes. When he was younger, he used to rock on his hands and knees, back and forth, rocking himself to sleep. Then he started jumping up and down.

HH—How is he in the morning when he wakes up?

Mother—Fine, in a good mood.

HH—What happens with him during sleep? Is he cold or perspiring, quiet in his sleep?

Mother—With four children, I sleep pretty good. When he wakes up, he's sweaty and wet. He does not like his hair washed or cut or his teeth brushed. He pitches a fit.

HH—How does he behave when you wash his hair?

Mother—Three months ago he started to scream, as if he's afraid I'm going to drown him.

HH—Can you tell us about your pregnancy? How was it compared with your others?

Mother—It wasn't near as much fun. He was born during July in Alabama. It was very hot and humid. I was 38 years old, swelled a lot, and had an amniocentesis. Normal pregnancy, no problems at the birth. Then, the next thing they told me was that he was in neonatal care. His color was bad, and they couldn't keep his temperature up. They couldn't tell us what was wrong, and we couldn't see anything wrong with him. His legs weren't getting good circulation, turning purple easily.

HH—Only in his legs?

Mother—Yes. I never noticed it in his arms.

HH—How was your mood during that pregnancy? We understand you weren't that happy in the beginning because it was a surprise. After that did you feel fine?

Mother—Yes.

HH—Was there any other special food craving in your pregnancy with him that was different from the others?

Mother—No. I don't remember anything special.

HH—Sleep was fine? Mood was okay? How about the amniocentesis?

Mother—The doctor insisted on it. He didn't tell me I had the option to say no.

HH—When did you discover you had that option?

Mother—After he was born.

HH—How about when you had the amniocentesis? Can you remember how he was behaving?

Mother—Everyone in the room said it was a boy: "He's doing great, in perfect position." Everything seemed to have gone fine.

HH—Did you follow his way of moving on the screen?

Mother—He seemed to be pretty calm.

HH—So he did not react to it?

Mother—No.

HH—How about his food?

Mother—He likes pasta, chicken noodle soup (a lot of soup), beans, no meat. I try to sneak the meat in. He'll pick around it in the soup. He eats ice cream, Popsicles, and junk.

HH—Is this his normal reaction to pain? [Child had fallen and bumped his head without much reaction to the bump.]

Mother—Yes.

HH—He screams for things he does not want, but not that much for pain?

Mother—No, not that much.

HH—He had breast milk in the beginning. How long?

Mother—Only a month. Having four children, every time I had to nurse him I was panicking. I breastfed the others, but I felt like I could not do this now.

HH—From the beginning?

Mother—Yes.

HH—How did he drink?

Mother—He did well, even in the hospital. For seven days, I nursed him every four hours. He did great.

HH—No difference between him and the other children?

Mother—No.

HH—When he was born, you saw him immediately? What was your impression of him?

Mother—He was my biggest at birth. He seemed fine; we were very happy. I thought he looked just like his dad. Four hours later, they came in with this problem. We couldn't believe it. We didn't understand, and they never found anything wrong with him. I was a little afraid, when I brought him home, that something might happen. My child before him didn't crawl. She scooted on her rear until she was two years old. When he was slow, I didn't think anything about it until about a year ago. I visited one of my three sisters, and one sister suggested I have him checked for autism. Little things seemed to be going in that direction. One psychologist thought at first that it was definitely autism, but then it seemed more like a developmental delay. He makes great eye contact and does not go into his own little world.

HH—How was your feeling toward the boy just after birth?

Mother—I don't remember right after birth, but when he was about three months old, I thought, "He's not responding when I looked at him. Not responding like the others did." He'd just sit there and watch us. He didn't react to us.

HH—At what age did he laugh?

Mother—That I don't remember.

HH—When did he walk?

Mother—At two years of age. He didn't crawl until after he was one year old.

HH—How did he react to hunger? Was he impatient?

Mother—No. When everyone else sits down, he gets in his chair, gets what he wants, takes the milk out. If I'm in the bathtub, he'll hand me the juice. He wants it put away immediately. He can get the soup he wants, hand it to me. He has to put it away immediately, does not want anything out of place. He likes slapping and clapping noises a lot.

HH—How is he in connection to his father?

Mother—He watches and knows about what time of day he comes home and is real excited. He jumps up and down and runs to the door to greet him. His dad likes to listen to music, and Kevin likes to dance and listen to music.

HH—Can you play with him?

Mother—Yes.

HH—What does he like to do?

Mother—Build with cardboard blocks, then knock them down. He likes to roll cars, play chase. He likes to play ball, but he won't roll it to me. He throws it in another direction so I have to go get it. His dad got him a battery-operated race car that scared me to death, but he was a whiz with it. He likes to write on himself. If he gets a pen, he'll write all over himself.

HH—He is a boy who is moving. Do you find him to be restless, moving around more than others his age?

Mother—No. Not more than other children. He is around a lot of children, and he is there amid them all. He does not like television as much as the others do.

HH—How does he react when it is on?

Mother—There has to be something that attracts his attention. He likes commercials. He acts like, "It's a commercial, I have to go. Good, good, good, good."

HH—He hasn't chosen, up to now, which is his favorite hand?

Mother—He uses a spoon with his right hand.

HH (to the child)—What are you making, Kevin? (No answer. He is drawing on the board, using either hand.)

Mother—He started at 18 months old saying, "Love." It stopped, but now he's saying other things; he does not say he loves anymore.

HH—If he is very happy, how does he express this happiness?

Mother—He laughs.

HH—Other ways?

Mother—He likes to flip the books. When he's happy, he does the rocking (when he's excited but not when he's unhappy).

HH—How about clothing?

Mother—Better than he used to be. He likes to have no clothes on at all. He'll wear them now, but usually the shirt goes first. Temperature makes no difference.

HH—He does not feel the cold that much?

Mother—I don't think so, because he does not react to it.

HH—How about his digestion? His stools?

Mother—He had a lot of problems with constipation when he was younger. Now he has hard pellets. He may not have a bowel movement every day.

HH—Does he go to the toilet himself, or do you use disposable diapers?

Mother—No. He will not go to the toilet. We've tried everything. Others told us to drain the water and paint targets. That didn't work either. But he likes to flush the toilet, especially while someone is still sitting there.

HH—How about understanding you when you speak to him?

Mother—When you ask him for a diaper, he goes to get it. Or he'll close the door or get something to eat when asked. He can say the names of his siblings. He screams when his sister closes the door in his face.

HH—He is silent and does not understand consequences?

Mother—Yes. If he wouldn't run into the street, it would be great.

HH—What is his mood usually? Describe it in one word.

Mother—Happy-go-lucky.

HH—He is not suffering in any certain way.

Mother—No.

HH—How does he react to pictures?

Mother—I show him family pictures. He looks behind them. He does not point or say who they are. He does not seem to recognize himself. (He is standing on his head with his butt up in the air.) A friend is at our house almost every day with a 16-month-old girl, and when she took his toys, he would take them back. Now she takes them back from him. He holds his own, and she does also. They kiss each other and hit each other, too.

HH—Let's go to the family history of health. We heard about your husband's family. How about your family's diseases?

Mother—I think that my father's mother lived to be in her mid-90s. His father died from heart trouble long before I was born. My mother's father died in his early 60s of skin cancer, and her mother died in her early 80s of breast cancer. My father has emphysema and is 76 years old. He's also an alcoholic. My mother is a hypochondriac and thinks everything's wrong with her, but she's in good health. My health is fine; my older sister has a thyroid condition. My other two sisters are fine.

HH—Anything else in particular about your son compared with your other children?

Mother—He likes to do everything they like to do, except that he likes to be outside more. He likes to play on the computer when they do. He likes to climb a lot.

HH—More than the other children?

Mother—I think so.

HH—Is there anything else he does not want to do that they wanted to do at his age?

Mother—No. He pretty much does what the other children do. In the airport today, several children were running around, and I couldn't tell that he was different from the others. He wants to get down from his chair to run in a restaurant. He runs for the door and screams.

_HH_—Is this the way he usually behaves?

Mother—This is it. If you confine him, he does not like it. When we go out, he's happy to go get in the car seat.

_HH_—When he fans himself with the pages of the book, do you think it is the touch of the paper he likes?

Mother—I don't know if it's the wind or the feel of the paper brushing his face.

_HH_—Does he like the wind outside?

Mother—No, not really.

_HH_—Most of the time he makes the paper touch him. How is he with touch, when you support him or when he is in your lap?

Mother—I have the impression that it is the touch of the book.

_HH_—How was he in the plane?

Mother—Good. He watched out the window, put the trays up and down. He was asleep for the landing.

_HH_—How is the color of his face most of the time? He is a little pale, with circles around his eyes.

Mother—He's usually a little bit pale. My other children are, too. We have a swimming pool, but they don't get sun.

_HH_—Does he have other habits except flipping the book pages and biting his clothes?

Mother—He used to rock on his hands and knees. He does not do that at all now. (He gets upset) mostly when he's tired, and he wants the books we won't let him have. He points to them and screams when he's sleepy. He likes to be tickled on his neck and his stomach. I play a little spider game, and then he does it to himself. He laughs and laughs. I sing "Old MacDonald" so many times that you'd think he would know it by now. (He climbs up on a chair but is still flipping the book.)

_HH_—I observe now that he is not making contact with anybody. Sometimes he can make contact with others?

Mother—He sucks his cheeks in a lot.

HH—How was his teething?

Mother—All came in on time. There didn't seem to be any problem. He does not like to have them brushed at all. My friend bathed her little one, and he screamed when she bathed him.

HH—How is his screaming?

Mother—Really high pitched.

HH—When he was drinking at the breast, what was your impression of him? I have the impression that every child nurses differently. (The mother thinks but does not seem to remember.)

Colleagues' Questions

[*He was two years old when he started to walk. Did he crawl normally?*]

Mother—Yes. Not until he was one. Before he crawled, he kind of rolled.

[*Sometimes when there are older siblings, the youngest does not have to talk. I'm wondering if he does not need to. Is it something more than that?*]

Mother—Yes. With the delay of everything else.

[*Was there any trauma in his young life, physical or otherwise?*]

Mother—(Shakes her head no.)

[*He was born and was with you. Then you went to have a tubal ligation, and until then he seemed fine?*]

Mother—I didn't think he looked abnormal.

[*Did you see that he looked purple?*]

Mother—I didn't see that; I could only see the IV and tubes. My sister went with me and said he was purple.

[*Was there any reaction to vaccinations?*]

Mother—No. He never ran a fever or anything like that. I've read that vaccinations at 18 months can cause inflammation of the brain. This is when it is often diagnosed, and they stop talking. The only thing that happened, as far as we know, is the blueness the first day after birth, for which he was given antibiotics. They started that before a doctor ever came. Then they did the sonogram of his heart, and his brain scan was normal. There was nothing. He just couldn't keep his color.

[*Did he get a vaccination in the hospital? In the state where I live, they automatically give a neonatal vaccine if you don't sign something.*]

Mother—I don't know that. They didn't circumcise him until the sixth day.

[*What was his reaction to that?*]

Mother—I don't think he acted differently from my other son.

[*If he had an Apgar score of 8 or 9, do you know what they deducted for?*]

Mother—They weren't concerned at all. He sucked very well right after birth.

[*How does he react to noises at home?*]

Mother—Only one time, when he had an ear infection, he would scream when we turned the vacuum on. He's never been on many antibiotics after that.

[*Can anyone else hold him like you do other than your husband?*] (She holds him close and rocks him.)

Mother—He does that with my husband, and a friend who is a bachelor, or my sisters.

[*When does he sleep?*]

Mother—He takes a nap for at least two hours. He still does not like to go to bed before 11:00 P.M., even after a nap, and likes to sleep until at least 10:00 A.M.

[*Childhood diseases?*]

Mother—He hasn't had any. My oldest two had chickenpox. He had a terrible diaper rash after the round of antibiotics at the hospital. The doctor gave me medication [cortisone cream that knocked the rash out], and the next day it was gone.

[*It was only on his bottom?*]

Mother—Yes.

[*Does he bite his fingernails or just suck on his sleeve?*]

Mother—No. Just on his sleeve.

HH—He gives me a lot of signs that show he may not be autistic. This is not how an autistic child behaves.

Mother—That's what I thought. He can make contact with other people. (He made quick contact with the video cameraman.)

Syphilis Case 2—Analysis

Can you imagine that the mother has a lot of problems with him? Was it from the vaccination? No. There was something already wrong at his birth because he had an Apgar score of 8. This was her fourth child, and he appeared to be fine. Then she said goodbye, went to the operating room, and his color got worse. The long cord was wrapped around him several times. Give some of your ideas as to what is happening with this child.

[*She had an epidural, which numbed the cervix. She said the epidural did not work; she felt the whole thing. Maybe it went into the bloodstream. It could have been a delayed reaction from that.*]

[***PH****—The mother is very strong, but she acquiesces to her husband easily. He thought the doctors just wanted to keep the baby in the hospital for the money. Also, she would hold him under the leg; and the leg would get blue there sometimes.*]

HH—There is a lack of memory in the mother's case about what happened in the first few hours with the baby. It is more usual to remember your child's birth very well. There was a reason I kept coming back to this point. Her sister noticed that the child was blue, but the mother did not see this. I find this a strange reaction. We see that the relationship is okay with her, but there is a kind of distance from the child. I observe this also when the child is playing around, when he is hitting his head. There is a mechanical calming down from the mother. I wondered whether on the stage it was because she had to behave in a certain way. [*He didn't make really good contact with me but liked to look at the camera.*] [*When he is flipping the pages across his face, he's either looking away blankly or into the book with his eyes crossed.*]

[***PH****—He does not really make contact. He wanders around, pushes his toys. The mother says he follows the other kids around, and he does run around, but he does not play with them. I was at his house a few weeks ago; his sister laid out a deck of cards on the floor. They wanted to play a card game. He took the cards and threw them away. I gave him his own set of cards, and he didn't want that. He wanted their cards and to be involved but not in the same way they were. He seems dreamy and can lie on the floor by himself, not in much need of anything.*]

HH—What is the most SRP symptom in this boy? [*To me it's the lack of contact.*] There is no contact. Why? We do not know exactly. He is not speaking. Is there weakness? Has there been a lack of oxygen? Could the weakness be due to that? There are some things we do not know, but we have to consider the possibilities. I am taking the vaccinations out of the case as a causation.

[*There are a lot of children who had his problems in the hospital, and they did not become blue.*]

HH—You have to consider several possibilities.

[*Lying on the cord could have caused hypoxia, but sometimes they can still recover at birth.*]

HH—We can consider that the cord around his neck three times could be suicidal for a baby at birth. Have you ever considered this? If you think of this, you see the syphilitic miasm. [*I thought about the cord around his neck as being due to the nurses' clumsiness.*]

HH—He had a sycotic cord. A six-foot long cord is excessive. We see a lot of the syphilitic miasm: He does not respond to heat or cold; does not feel; is not sensitive; his left foot is turned in.

[*The page-turning is obsessive/compulsive. I thought at first it was a desire to be fanned. Now it seems to be a desire to be touched by the paper.*] [*He did repetitive actions, opening and shutting the door, putting things away.*]

[*Especially for somebody who does not notice things going on around him.*]

HH—If his mother takes the milk out and puts it in the wrong cup, he grunts for another cup. He pours it from one to another. He does it very carefully. His depth perception wasn't good. His mother said he laughs when his father cracks the ice. The child knows how to express himself. He wanted to go out. He has his own way of expressing it. He is better outside.

[*He likes to see things moving—commercials, water pouring, words on the screen.*]

HH—He wants action. For example, I have a patient who is slow in action but what he draws is only airplanes—always airplanes. All he cares about is planes. He finds his speed in his drawings of airplanes. This is a compensation for his slowness.

At his age, he should have fear of falling. He has fallen down several times during the consultation, but shows no fear of falling. He was a little late developing the fear of getting his hair washed. This is usually at about one-and-a-half years of age. I do not think a healthy child has fear of animals unless he has gone through a bad experience. Precocious children sometimes develop fears of certain figures or wolves (usually around four years old), after the time when they start being told fairy tales. He does not react to animals at all. When he put the pencils on the floor, one fell down, and he liked the experience of something falling. This usually happens before the child is one year old. Due to this childishness, I am not surprised he cannot speak. He is developmentally too young.

[*Most babies need other people. He does not seem to need anyone other than to serve his needs.*]

HH—He has probably remained in the stage where he got into trouble. We must consider this as a sign as to why he could not develop.

Other Problems To Consider

- Apgar scores
- Amniocentesis
- Mother's edema during pregnancy
- Mother leaving for operating room and baby turns blue
- Vaccinations
- Panic of mother during pregnancy
- Father/family alcoholism

[*Some things weren't said about what the mother felt during the time she found out about the pregnancy. Maybe the husband wasn't happy about it. Maybe something wasn't said about it?*]

HH—This we don't know. It was more like "business as usual." When she told about doing something recently, I felt that there was something else going on that was not expressed. I was happy to see her toward the end of the consultation as a totally loving mother (holding the child on her lap when he got tired.) There is something that we see or feel in the mother, a tension, perhaps a sense of distance, or perhaps she is nervous in front of so many people.

[***PH***—*She is a loving mother with him. I've seen her in a lot of situations. She's always there for her children. When the baby was in intensive care, she went home and came back every four hours. The mother has smoked marijuana, but she's not an addictive personality. Her husband is, though. He uses alcohol every day until he goes to sleep. Both smoke cigarettes. I know she smoked before and after the pregnancy. She did not know she was pregnant, and so she probably smoked during the first months.*]

[*She breastfed the other children but did not continue to breastfeed this one. This is some indication that something was wrong.*]

[*He had an aversion to meat.*]

HH—I find this aversion to meat quite normal in children. Most little children do not particularly like meat. I find it unusual when they do. He does not eat bread, but he likes pasta. I do not think he is abnormally small, but he has a very fine face.

[*He didn't have much expression, but he laughed much at the camera.*]

Family History Summary

- Grandparents are all living.
- Dad's father has ulcers.
- Strong history of asthma in the family.
- Great-grandfather was probably a functioning alcoholic.
- Cancer in both families.

Discussion

Lack of contact can be syphilitic. The cord around his neck three times could be syphilitic or psoric. His left foot being turned in is syphilitic. Compulsive behavior can be syphilitic or psoric or even sycotic. Why? It is "overdoing"—doing the same things again and again. It is something he does when he needs to be doing better things, so this could be syphilitic. If it is for comfort, it could be psoric.

He loves running water. There is water in his history—the pouring, getting the can of soup out of the cabinet. This could be tubercular or sycotic due to the movement. He's better outside and likes to run away. This could be tubercular or sycotic. He stays up late—sycotic or tubercular—and perhaps syphilitic when there is a kind of flatness about going to bed. He wakes refreshed—psoric or maybe tubercular. Chewing on his sleeves—a kind of contact, and for comfort. This could be psoric. It could be syphilitic if they bite their clothes instead of chewing the food they need.

What about shrieking? He has this during fear and when he wants something. This could be psoric, tubercular, or syphilitic (children need to ask instead of shrieking). I have a granddaughter who is one-and-a-half years old, who points to things when she does not know a word. She does not have to shriek. When I do not know a word in English, I do not start to shriek.

What is lack of fear—psoric, syphilitic, or tubercular? [*Psoric?*] Why psoric? His fear was not developed as a baby. It could also be sycotic. His lack of reaction could be psoric, syphilitic, sycotic, or tubercular.

Who likes soup? People too weak to chew. It is easier to get the food into the child when the food is cooked in small pieces. It is not laziness on his part because he is chewing his sleeve. Why can he not chew meat or bread? In Europe, most little children will chew the inside of the bread and put aside the crust because it is hard. Eating no meat is quite normal, but bread is one of the first forms of nourishment. Maybe it is childishness, which could be psoric.

How about blueness in newborns? What could be the reason? If it is because his mother left him after delivery, it could be psoric. We have almost every miasm in this case.

Symptom	**Miasm**
No contact, worse being looked at	Syphilitic
Late development	Syphilitic, psoric
Cord around neck three times	Syphilitic, psoric
Excessively long cord	Sycotic
Left foot turned in	Syphilitic
Compulsive behavior	Can be all
Water—likes to see it running	Tubercular, sycotic
Better outside	Tubercular, sycotic
Stays up late	Sycotic, tubercular, syphilitic
Wakes refreshed	Psoric, tubercular
Chews his sleeve	Psoric, syphilitic
Shrieking	Psoric, tubercular, syphilitic
Lack of fear	Psoric, tubercular, syphilitic
Backward, slow development, childish	Psoric, tubercular, syphilitic
Lack of reaction (does not feel cold or heat)	Psoric, tubercular, syphilitic, sycotic
Blueness—newborn	Psoric, tubercular

In *Kent's Repertory* we have the rubric: **RESPIRATION; ASPHYXIA; *newborn infant*** (8): **Ant-t.**, **Camph.**, *arn.*, *bell.*, *laur.*, *op*, acon., chin. Let's look at some of the remedies in this rubric and consider their sensitivity to pain and touch.

- *Arnica* [*feels "There is nothing wrong with my baby; he's fine."*]
- *Camphora* [*coldness*]
- *China* [*likes little things to touch him*]. How is China about touch? They like hard touch and not soft touch. He loves little things.

- *Laurocerasus* [*they are cold and blue, and have lack of reaction—are happy outside, have mental dullness, and heavy sleep, weakness of rectum and runny stools*]
- *Opium* [*painlessness*]
- *Antimonium tartaricum* is one of the remedies in this rubric. Might our patient need this remedy? We would have a history of mucus, which is not there.

Look also at another rubric in *Kent's Repertory*: **GENERALITIES; CYANOSIS; *infants, in*** (17): **Dig.**, **Lach.**, **Laur.**, *bor.*, *cact.*, *camph.*, *carb-v.*, *naja*, *phos.*, arn., ars., chin., op., psor., rhus-t., sec., sulph.

- *Borax*? [*No. He loves to run down things. Downward motion is against Borax.*]
- *Carbo vegetabilis?* [*wants his face fanned*]
- *Digitalis*? [*He has heart irregularity.*] [*They have fear of dying if they stop moving.*] They have a lot of guilty feelings.
- *Lachesis*? [*Our patient is better on waking in the morning, and he does not talk.*]
- *Phosphorus?* [*would be making contact*]
- *Psorinum*? [*He has no skin symptoms.*]

When we go through these rubrics, we have two possible remedies: *Arnica* and *Laurocerasus*. I want you to take this case as homework. Think about the case tonight as well as about these two remedies. The mother insisted that there was nothing wrong with her child. We still see this type of reaction in her. [*Does Laurocerasus have this mental problem, too?*] It can have. Read *Laurocerasus* tonight. Look at childishness, lateness learning to walk or talk, chewing his sleeve, rubrics for shrieking, and lack of fear.

Discussion of Yesterday's Case

Did you study the case from yesterday? Who studied these two remedies, or who has a new remedy? [*I still feel Opium is a good choice.*] [*I thought of Sepia because of the stasis.*] What also favors *Sepia*? [*The mother's distance, his running, his indifference to people.*] [*He was insistent on what he wanted without concern for others.*] *Sepia* is mostly sycotic, a little psoric, and not much syphilitic.

Other remedies that came out? [*Mercurius. I repertorized "Naked, wants to be," "Impulse to touch things," and "Rocking." It was strong in a couple of these rubrics.*] It is also syphilitic (his not making much contact), and he has restlessness. [*Tuberculinum: desire for fresh air, paleness, blueness, and demand for what he wants.*]

Did anyone study *Arnica* and *Laurocerasus*? **What is in favor or not in favor of *Arnica*?** [*It is listed as a cold remedy in the literature. They have an aversion for soup, touch aggravates them, sleep aggravates, and movement aggravates.*] And they have a lot of fears. They do have the feeling they are okay, and we have the emotional trauma of the child. [*Arnica has mind symptoms and cardiac symptoms from anguish and fear of death with cardiac symptoms.*] Yes, there are wonderful rubrics that tell how an *Arnica* patient can get heart problems when there is an emotional problem. We have a very strong symptom. The causation could also fit *Arnica.*

What is in favor of *Laurocerasus*? [*They were incredibly similar when we compared the mind symptoms only. We had to go to "Generalities" to individualize the remedies. And Laurocerasus is a small remedy compared to Arnica.*] [*When I see Laurocerasus patients in the hospital, they seem to be fine when born, and then suddenly they aspirate or turn blue. It reminds me of how this patient was.*]

Before the baby sucked the breast, there was something wrong with him; and we do not know what it was. When I think logically about what happened, the mother got an anesthetic, which did not help. In a few hours, she had to undergo surgery again. It is awful to do two things like this in the same day. The mother is tired from labor, then she has the stress that the narcotic does not work. When the mother had to undergo the second surgery and it did not work, I am sure the child drank in her emotional feelings. There is a lot we do not know exactly, but we have some facts. She kissed the baby goodbye, went for surgery, had narcotics, and came back to the shock of having her baby in intensive care. She breastfed the baby, went home, came back, went home, and came back. As soon as he went home and she tried to feed him, she felt panic. There are a lot of things the mother has gone through, and the baby went through these, too. It is not easy to decide which remedy in this case.

There are things a little contrary to the case. The mother thought, "My baby is well; there is nothing the matter." We know that, after that time, she worried all the time about the baby. The two remedies have a lot in common in the mental sphere, but not the fear. The fear is much more pronounced in *Arnica.* How about modalities: cold, heat, motion? [*In Laurocerasus it said that they never recover from the initial problem. It takes a long time for improvement. He seems to be still in that state.*] *YES! THIS IS IMPORTANT!* He did not grow. There was a moment in his life that stopped him from growing.

How does *Arnica* look? She (the mother) has a red face. [*Laurocerasus is pale to blue. He has a little bluish tint around his eyes.*] [*Arnica does not want to be touched and neither does Laurocerasus.*] [*He wants to tickle himself.*] Yes, he wants to touch himself, which is against *Arnica.* We know many rubrics that show that *Arnica* is sensitive to touch and aggravated by touch, but this is not strong in *Laurocerasus.* He is not worse from strong touch. When he bumped his head, his first reaction was for Mom to rub it. I like it when these spontaneous things happen during an interview. The idea of touch is against *Arnica.* The asphyxia and thinking there is nothing wrong with her baby are pro-*Arnica.* How about the desire to be outside? *Arnica* does not want to be outside. *Laurocerasus* is ameliorated by fresh air.

Miasmatically, *Laurocerasus* is syphilitic, psoric, and tubercular. When you look at heart problems and respiration problems after birth, *Laurocerasus* comes up more strongly. [*Clarke's Materia Medica says about Laurocerasus, "She could not articulate for the thickness and heaviness of the tongue."*] [*Laurocerasus has a forsaken feeling, which fits the idea of his being separated from his mother just after birth.*] [*We saw an impulsive quality in him, and in Kent's Repertory I found Laurocerasus under "Impetuous" but did not find Arnica.*]

Symptom	**Arnica**	**Laurocerasus**
TOUCH	<Touch	Touch can agg. though not strongly
OUTSIDE	<Outside	>Outside
FEARS	<Being touched	<Being forsaken
SLEEP	<Sleep	>Sleep
COLOR	Red face	Blueness
RESPONSE	"I'm OK"	Forgets to speak
MOVEMENT	Restless	Restless
TIME	Weakness A.M.	Relaxed in A.M.

It was added later to other repertories, but what is strongest in this child: refusal to answer or the impetuous quality we saw in him that could be like

Arnica? Is *Arnica* impulsive? In a certain way, when there has been an accident and she is lying on the floor. Someone asks how she is, and she says, "I am fine." This is a kind of impulsiveness, but since that accident, *Arnica* will be fearful. She will be stuck in the idea that she has to run away from any accident. In other ways, our patient is not very impulsive. I see that he wanted to go outside, but I wasn't sure he was impulsive. [*He knew what he did, bringing the book to his face. Laurocerasus is also listed under* **MIND; THOUGHTS; *persistent*.**]

The modalities and generalities characteristic in this case are against *Arnica*. The pathology at the moment something happened is more strongly found in *Laurocerasus*. If you ever have to treat the mother of this child, we see strong indications for two possible remedies: *Sepia* and *Arnica*.

The nice thing is that we don't see *Laurocerasus* that often. I have seen a *Laurocerasus* colleague who was unable to study homeopathy. In her case, by seeing others she could learn it; and she is a good homeopath. However, it was impossible for her to read. She could learn only by observing in seminars. She knew she needed help to study better. One of her shoulders was dislocated during her birth, and was lame for several months as a little child. During stress, she felt her shoulder problem again. Her mother had told her, "Be happy it was only your shoulder because you were almost dead. You were blue." One of her modalities was liking to be outside because she could think better outside. She could think of her cases while walking in the fresh air, and then she could get the remedies in her mind. *Laurocerasus* unlocked her case.

[*You gave the symptom of blueness a lot of weight. Can you explain?*]

I used the rubric, **GENERALITIES; CYANOSIS (74)** because a baby at birth is usually pink, maybe a little wrinkled. When he is blue, something is happening. His blueness went on. The mother said his legs became blue when she held him. We have the Apgar score, and I am sure the doctors are good at this, but I feel something is missing here. Most feel that an Apgar of 8 is okay. It is a technical diagnosis, measured carefully, but we know there was blueness. Blueness runs throughout the case.

It was strange that he did not speak because he has a certain cleverness. He is backward but able to do things. There is something blocking him. Something happened in his life that blocked him. The two things I can see are the incident after four hours and the birth itself, which was a strange one. [*I thought an Apgar score of 8 or 9 was excellent.*] To me, a child without problems should have a score of 10. [standard is 9.] When you have experience with patients, you will see quickly where the case started. There is a kind of logic you can see. If it is something that happened once, it is not that important. When you see repetition, this is important.

This boy does not have *Opium* symptoms. He is not sleepy at all. We only have the fact that he does not talk. If we know he needed *Laurocerasus* and he had been given the remedy at the age of five days, what would have been the difference? He would have developed in a normal way. Now we have the privilege of treating him at three-and-a-half years old. If he is not treated now, he would need to be taken care of his whole life. Better that he is treated now. He is backward, but he will grow quicker than normal in the emotional sphere. When he is 12 or 14 years of age, there may be no strong difference between him and other children. I would like to give him *Laurocerasus* 10M. Do you agree?

We had a case in our practice of a mother treated years ago for allergic reactions. In one year, she had two doses of *Lycopodium* and was fine. The homeopath saw her some weeks ago, and the mother was eight months pregnant. She had a pain in her right sinus, exactly like her allergic state some years ago. *Lycopodium* 200C was prescribed. She phoned the next day, saying her pain was much better. Three or four days later, this homeopath came into the kitchen, hysterical. She told me that two days after *Lycopodium*, the mother discovered the baby did not move anymore. The gynecologist discovered that the baby was dead. The homeopath thought she had killed the baby. My conclusion was that the baby was already dead, and therefore the mother got her old allergic symptom back in a cry for help. I consoled the homeopath, telling her that homeopathy could not kill the baby. I told her that I was sure she had prescribed the right remedy and that something was going on before this last prescription. Three days later, the homeopath came in with a smile and said that she got the autopsy report. The baby had been dead three days before the remedy. The cord was wrapped around his neck; he died in utero. Life is very strong, and to kill with a homeopathic remedy would be very strange.

Syphilis Case 2—Followup

Kevin has been seen in seminar for four years. He has had one repetition of *Laurocerasus* 10M in the four years since his initial remedy in January

2000. The repeat was given after the child had received antibiotics for bronchitis. It is possible that he did not need the repeat of the remedy at that time, but his present homeopath is impatient, wanting more changes to occur more quickly than she sees.

The remedy works like a top: If you touch it while it is spinning, it stops. You cannot make it go any faster or any better without stopping its action. You have to wait until it stops by itself.

Thinking we can do something to make the remedy work faster and better is allopathic thinking. This child progresses slowly, but definitely.

The first year after the remedy he became a little more alert, a subtle change. I cautioned the mother that, if he should develop an illness, he should not be given any medication but that she should contact the homeopath. When the child developed a fever in May (16 months after his initial remedy), antibiotics were given. The remedy was repeated, and the child continued to improve slowly. Within the following eight months, there were more visible improvements. During the first 16 months, the remedy was working at a deep level where we could not see it. He was seen again in January 2002, and I again cautioned the mother not to treat him with any medication should he develop an acute illness. The illness would come only when he was stronger, and after such an illness, by recovering on his own, or with his remedy if needed, he would become much stronger.

Who can see illness? We cannot see illness; we can only see its manifestations in symptoms.

Do we see the whole illness? No, we only see a few of the symptoms that are given to us by the patient (or parents) in the consultation. There may be other symptoms that he does not tell you about, either because he thinks they are normal or because he does not want to talk about them. When the patient returns for followup and you review the list of his symptoms, he may say there is no change in any of them, but when you ask about other things, he says, for example, that his colleagues are much friendlier now. If you are a beginner, you may think the remedy is not working, but something has changed in his way of feeling. Later, the physical symptoms will change, because right now his energy has gone into his behavior, to fix that.

Before Kevin's followup in January 2003, I met the child and his mother in the lobby on my way to lunch. The child looked up at me and said, "Hi, Henny." I looked at his homeopath and said, "This is your reward for waiting." The child had developed another fever in the summer, and the mother remembered the caution not to treat him. His fever lasted one day and one night. One week later he began to speak in full sentences. He has become much more connected to himself and his family, is in school, is reading, and is memorizing lines for his play. He is in a martial arts class and is able to participate and follow instructions like the other children in the class. The parents feel that these tiny white pills have given them back their son who was blocked at birth.

Prescribe Only When Necessary

Do you see why you must not give remedies for every minor complaint? Be aware of your patients saying, "No change." I think we lack respect for our own work. Take time to let your patients go through the treatment when you are treating them chronically. Caution them not to change homeopaths quickly; your patients can prevent the healing work of your remedy because they do not see changes fast enough or in the way they anticipate.

I once treated an autistic boy who got the right remedy, came out of his autistic state, started to play, got an old ear inflammation back, was treated with antibiotics, and then went back to the autistic state. We repeated the remedy, and he got the ear infection again. I had warned the parents to contact me when this happened. They did, and I told them not to do anything. I said, "Phone me tomorrow." The next day, the pain was gone, and the eardrum erupted. The child was okay and could take a painkiller. A discharge started from his ear the next day. Again, I had told them to contact me. They called and asked, "How long will this last?" The father said, "My mother tells me I am a fool to go to a homeopath." I told them to wait. Better to have a child with a deaf ear than a child who is autistic. I felt they weren't accepting this, so I told them to phone me the next day. However, there were no more phone calls. Two months later, I was to see the boy in front of a big group. I saw him in the corridor shouting, crying, and more autistic than before. When I saw the father, I said, "What did you do?" He said, "I gave him only two spoonfuls of antibiotics." The child was worse than before. It took a long time to get him out of this situation. He had a very weak vital force. I told them, "If you suppress again, there will be trouble." Be aware of doing things in so-called "acute situations."

What is an "acute situation?" [*A manifestation of the chronic.*] For example, you treat someone for emphysema, and after the correct remedy, he gets bronchitis. What do you have to do? Nothing. He is moving toward a cure. If he does not improve, you may have to interfere with the remedy. But why change remedies if the remedy picture is the same?

This is what makes it difficult to do homeopathy—that little allopathic voice we all have in our minds. We are tempted to think this way even if we have done homeopathy for years. We always want to try this or that. You have to sit down quietly, take a deep breath, and take the case. Do not be afraid of acting in a homeopathic way.

If the theory is true for the chronic treatment of patients, which should we rely on: our allopathic worries or the teachings of the old masters?

Apply the Miasms

Sometimes we hesitate in our prescriptions during chronic treatment because we see a remedy come forward that we are unsure of. What remedy do you prescribe? [*The indicated remedy.*] Of course, even when it is *Nux moschata* or *Cannabis indica.*

Let's say our patient is a very young boy with aggression. We give him *Mercurius.* He comes back when he is 18 years old and we see the same state we saw in the beginning, but this time without the disposable diapers and the bottle. Let's say his problems started after an accident when he was given antibiotics or after cocaine use or an LSD trip. He was all right before, but now he has hysteria, a dry mouth, and a *Nux moschata* picture. You go back in his history, and you see that he has some symptoms that before looked like *Mercurius.* What should you do? If you give *Mercurius* at this time, it will not work—just as *Pulsatilla* would not have helped him originally.

If you see that the patient was in a particular state at one time but that now there is a clear picture of another state, you must give the remedy for the present state. After the work of the correct remedy, the second state will come out wonderfully.

Then you prescribe the miasmatic remedy needed, and it will clear the case. Apply the miasms. It makes your homeopathy easier.

CHAPTER 3

Sycosis and the Sycotic Miasm

The sycotic miasm is the result of suppressed gonorrhea. Sycosis has its origin in the fig wart, the wart that can be contracted after someone has sexual intercourse with a person who has gonorrhea. Here again, there is something in the sycotic miasm that is in contrast to the psoric miasm. We know that psora and its miasm were well established in the early history of human beings. We all have psora, regardless of circumstances, because our ancestors all had psora. But for our ancestors to get the disease of syphilis or gonorrhea, the choice of the sexual act was decisive. The will became involved. One had to choose to do something. In psora, the will was not involved.

Where there is sycosis there is also the base of psora. Hahnemann said that when sycotic symptoms are strong and prominent, we must give a sycotic remedy first, then the psoric miasm will come out.

How does sycosis get into the life of a person? It can come from suppressed gonorrhea in the patient or in family members (e.g., father, mother, grandparents). Moreover, if a healthy psoric woman marries a sycotic man, she may develop cystitis, pain in the ovaries, or a vaginal discharge. Even when this sycotic husband does not have gonorrhea, his psoric wife may develop sycotic complaints from their sexual contact because he is carrying the miasm of his ancestry, and miasms can spread through sexual contact, even without an active sexual infection. The psoric wife normally will not develop the emotional and mental symptoms of sycosis; rather, she may complain of physical discomfort or pain in the lower abdomen, which begins after sexual contact with her sycotic husband. When there is a history of "before the marriage I was fine," we must, of course, treat the woman, but also try to treat her husband.

Another way to establish the presence of the sycotic miasm is through vaccinations in the patient or a family history of vaccinations. A vaccination touches one's miasmatic possibilities. When vaccinations cause certain reactions such as a sudden high fever, swelling, redness, heat, and hyperactivity, the sycotic miasm has been touched, and the patient will need a sycotic remedy, not simply because he has had the vaccination, but because of his reaction to the vaccination. We know *Thuja* as a strongly sycotic remedy that can help overcome problems that may result from vaccinations. Not everyone responds to vaccination with a sycotic reaction. If one develops an itch, it shows a psoric reaction. Meningitis after vaccination is a syphilitic reaction.

Mental and Emotional Symptoms and Expressions of the Sycotic Miasm

Excess—too much—overabundance
Liveliness
Expressive
Loves celebrations/parties/fun
Fast/hurried
Impatient
Boastful
High-energy
Strength and endurance
Tendency to overdo
Ameliorated by movement
Loves nightlife
Goes to extremes
Exaggerates
Exuberant
Outgoing
Jealous
Impulsive
Erratic
Has strong polarities
Loves animals

One can feel the difference in the nature and energy of the sycotic miasm just by reading the list of words we use to describe it. Where there was weakness in psora, now there is power. Where there was a quiet, shy reserve in psora, now there is flashy exuberance. What is important to understand is how this influence affects the health of our patients.

The active sycotic miasm is about **too much** and **extremes**. When we first see a patient in the waiting room, we get some clues about him. We can recognize the different miasms in the patient's outlook and demeanor. When sycosis comes into the waiting room, it is marvelous. The waiting room starts to come alive. The sycotic patient is so **outgoing** that he talks to everyone. A tip for our practices: We homeopaths can plan the energy of our office waiting room by filling our appointment slots with not just one kind of patient, but with a variety of miasms.

When the sycotic patient tells us her complaints, she is not shy. She is **expressive**. She may stand up and point out every symptom, no matter where in her body. She can seem to fill the room.

Although psora may live a long life with much complaining, sycosis has fun all his life—talking, celebrating, and having sex. He may not complain, he may feel quite strong, yet his heart can become **enlarged** because of his sycosis, and he can die at 55 years of age. Once, when I expressed these ideas to a class, a student came to me after the lecture and said he preferred to be a sycotic. Why? "Better a happy short life than complaining all my life."

Even little babies show their expressions of psora, sycosis, or syphilis. The trick is to know what we are seeing. While the psoric child will walk or be carried into the homeopath's office, the sycotic child will run or jump because sycosis does everything faster. There is **hurriedness and impatience** in sycosis, rather than the slower plodding of psora.

Sycosis likes **excess and excitement**. He is extroverted and exuberant and likes to show off. Sycosis buys **flashy** cars with six speakers that play loud music—the music can be heard three to five miles away. Or he might buy a van so he can pick up all of his friends, drive them around, and have drinking parties in the van. We must always be looking for the clues that will help us truly understand what is going on in our patients. Sycosis **likes company**. He will use alcohol to have a good time. "Let's all drink and have **fun**." A sycotic entertains; he remembers and tells us all about his many parties.

Miasmatic influence can be recognized in every choice we make. Does the sycotic influence persuade one to buy a small breed of dog? Probably not. Generally, sycosis will buy a dog that is large and energetic—he considers this type a "real dog," not a toy. Sycosis likes animals because they give excitement, because one can be **active** with animals. One can ride a horse very fast and jump with it. With a dog, one can show who is master. Sycotic men like to show they are macho. Men who want to build up big muscles to show off and be "tough" have a sycotic mental state. Sycosis can be a big **boaster**.

Sycosis also can be **dictatorial** and **bossy**. We all know people who are domineering, hurried, and impatient. Sycosis will say, "I need or want this *right now*" or "You need to do it for me *immediately*." Sycosis feels that his needs come first. When someone imposes himself on another, this is clearly the sycotic miasm. Sycosis exhibits haughtiness because he feels he is the best. A woman who wants to draw attention to herself may think, "I will only marry a man with a limousine" (a sycotic kind of car) or "I will marry a prince or someone who is rich." This is the **ostentation** of sycosis.

Sycosis prefers to live in town rather than in the country. Cities and towns are exciting—people, noise, music, entertainment, smells. She likes to be with people at parties, dancing. She **makes connections** with other people easily because she is outgoing. The connections may be superficial, but she will never isolate herself as syphilis does.

People often choose professions that allow them, in some way, to express their needs, confront their fears, or compensate for their state. Sycosis may choose a profession with an element of **excitement**, **stimulation**, or **action**—perhaps sales, because in sales there is stimulation in meeting people—a successful outlet for their outgoing, forward nature. Sycosis usually chooses a career that involves taking risks. He might become an **entertainer**. He does not want to sit at a steady, stable job with rules as does psora. Because of his need for movement and his **strength, high energy, and power**, he might choose to play professional sports or engage in excessive sport or strong physical labor. Surely it will be a job with a lot of exhilaration or physical effort.

Sycosis loves **nightlife** and craves more and more. When we give sycosis a stimulant, he cannot stop himself; he goes on and on. Sycotic people prefer loud, fast music with a strong beat. When some young people go to a disco on Friday evening, they bring fresh shirts. They start dancing, and when they are covered in sweat they go to the car, change clothes and go back in. They dance from Friday evening to Monday morning until the disco closes. In a town close to where I live, one disco now reopens on Monday at 7:00 A.M. and stays open until that afternoon for those who weren't satisfied with only the weekend! The owner of the disco says his best business is on Monday morning. These are the sycotic youngsters. Some even supplement their experience with Ecstasy pills. Fun, excitement, nightlife, people, movement—this is the energetic pattern of the sycotic remedy *Medorrhinum.*

Sycosis can work into the night because she has lots of **energy**; the later it gets, the better she feels. She constantly wants to do things. She is restless and **sleepless from excitement**, not from anxiety like psora or from suffering and misery like syphilis. Sycosis might say, "The only way to get to sleep is to switch on the radio and dance for a while." The more typical thing to do when you cannot fall asleep is to try to be peaceful, in quiet, dark surroundings, so that your mind and body slow down and you can rest into sleep.

Sycosis is excited in the night, **stays up late**, and is not very good in the morning. She may feel tired and weak. She likes to sleep during the day. Her dreams may include sexual activity, dancing, and enjoying life. She may talk and laugh in her sleep and wake often. Her mind is **overstimulated**.

The sycotic miasm is energetic. He can cope for a long time. His energy can be quite **strong**. He can stay up late at night, and although it may be difficult, can get up the next morning and start again. He can tolerate a lot of what would be energetically stressful for psora. He can be quite active, using a lot of energy all the time and not really feel the excess. There is activity in the tubercular miasm, too, but the overactive energy of tuberculosis does not have as much **endurance** as the energy of sycosis. Sycosis will do things such as aerobics, running and jumping, and dancing to loud music—moving, doing many things at the same time. Sycosis can get energy by doing these things. When someone with a sycotic background runs a race, he will win. He has to win; he needs to win. He may start to dance and not be able to stop for hours. This is the "too much" of sycosis.

In sycosis there is a need to **move**. He needs to move even when he is ill because he is better from movement; he cannot be still. He will often do more than is reasonable. His mind may feel chaotic, with too much thinking. He is not able to make a decision or to focus, not out of weakness, but because there is so much happening at once in him. He may do many things in a short time and be unable to finish any of them.

Nothing is too dangerous or too quick for sycosis. He goes to **extremes**. He exercises too much. He likes action. He likes speed racing and bungee jumping—sports with excessive risk taking. He chooses these activities not to hurt himself, but because of the thrill, the excitement, the fun. He feels invincible.

Sycosis is "open" and independent. Psora will ask for support, but sycosis will find a way out by acting and doing. The behavior of sycosis is comparable to that period in puberty when young people are rebellious—wanting adventure, testing their limits, not doing what their parents tell them to do but finding their own way and getting into their own trouble. During puberty, we feel we want to get away, travel to other countries, and do new things. Young (and older) people who live only for the next adventure, for the highest excitement, are sycotic. They do not worry about the future. They do things NOW.

There is sycotic behavior in **excessive** talking. Sycosis talks as an outlet—loquacity. She has to get things out, to discharge.

Sycosis is **impulsive, erratic, and changeable**. He'll decide in a moment, "I will leave my wife and children because I have found the religion of my life." These tendencies can be seen on an individual basis and even in groups of people.

In general, sycosis has little fear—except perhaps of being bored. If she has fear, she will deal with it in a sycotic way. She will either confront her fear by becoming involved in what she fears—as when *Thuja* decides to climb a mountain, or when *Argentum nitricum* takes a job as an elevator operator—or she will run away to escape it. Either way, she **responds quickly**. Psora, however, usually avoids dealing with her fears; instead, she worries. Syphilis complains about all the things he does not like and how bad the world is; he gets depressed. **Sycosis overreacts quickly and with energy**.

When sycosis feels anger, he experiences strong outbursts, and then the anger is over. He has "fits" of anger—perhaps shouting, telling someone how he feels, releasing and **discharging quickly**—and then he feels better. If he feels he cannot act to release the anger, he runs away to avoid or escape the problem. Sycosis reacts "on the spot" by reacting immediately. His anger must surface in some action, and then it goes away quickly. When the sycotic homeopath is stumped by a case, he might shout and curse. He has little patience for reviewing a case carefully He prefers to have a quick consultation, with a quick repertorization, and decide the remedy in 10 minutes. He may shout and curse when he discovers that someone has borrowed one of his treatment books and has not returned it, but he gets over it.

Mania with rage and **increased strength** are sycotic. Sycosis is the fighting miasm. For example, a sycotic symptom in *Causticum* is to fight an injustice. Sycosis will fight after the death of someone close to her. If a *Causticum* woman's child dies in a car accident from the driver's alcohol abuse, she will initiate and organize, or join a group such as Mothers Against Drunk Driving, and fight to prevent this from happening again.

Action, speed, and sex are what sycosis looks for and enjoys in movies. She gets excited about movies with guns and blood, and if she should get the impulse to kill, it will be in some state of excitement or jealousy—not because of hatred with the desire to kill. She likes to read novels about someone who runs away with friends and has an adventure or a party.

Sycosis likes **strong bright colors**—red, yellow, and orange—and often will dress in these colors. You cannot miss him. He shows his body, accentuating his sexual attributes. Women who are sycotic use bright red lip coloring. Of course, homeopaths do not prescribe on colors, but colors often fit into the picture. People undergo body piercing (self-mutilation) for different reasons. Sycosis does it to shock others and be noticed.

One aspect of sycosis is a kind of **shamelessness**, with a high sex drive—too much, too early, and too fast. When sycosis has a headache, he may want sex to feel better. In the consulting room, sometimes patients exhibit symptoms without even knowing it. Sycosis might say, "Hi, sweetheart." He will touch and kiss everybody. The need to grasp and pinch is sycotic.

Sycosis is very **spontaneous** and impulsive about telling things. She likes to tell jokes with a sexual connotation. At celebrations, she is the one surrounded by others who are sycotic, exchanging sexual jokes. She cannot hide her sycotic feelings. Cursing, lewd talk, and ribald jokes are all sycotic. Jesting and practical jokes also are sycotic.

One of my patients with epilepsy had an aura just before he experienced a seizure. He went to his neighbor's home, where he undressed himself and then had the seizure. This is sycotic behavior. When giving his case, he remembered he had gone to the neighbor's, but he did not know he had undressed. In the consulting room, this man was shocked when his wife mentioned this. However, I remembered that on his first visit he entered my consulting room and said to me, "Hey, my little pussycat." This was sycotic.

Sycosis likes a lot of sex, more for the **stimulation** and the excitement than for the emotional contact. She does not like the perverted sex of syphilis, but she enjoys sex and movement—sexual gymnastics. Dressing and behaving provocatively, sexual exposure, touching the genitals, and wanting to be naked are sycotic. Yet, too much constant sexual activity and indulgence can wear sycosis down. The homeopath may see sycosis in a state of decline after her energy is depleted. A 50-year-old sycotic can be broken down and impotent. If the homeopath suspects that he is sycotic, he or she should ask how he was before this worn-out state, which will reveal the energy of sycosis.

Although sycosis is very sexual, rape is violent and therefore syphilitic. Sycosis **tries to hide** what he feels are the bad parts of his behavior, but in most things he shows himself and celebrates everything with lots of music and sound. When a sycotic person lies, it is possible that he is trying to hide bad behavior, but he can also lie for the fun of it, for the thrill of tricking us or exaggerating.

When sycosis is **jealous**, he will scream and shout, curse, or throw things, showing his jealousy. Or perhaps he will compete or overreact in some way. A sycotic woman who is jealous of her husband's secretary may begin flirting with other men to get her husband's attention. Sycosis may plot to get her boyfriend back or take revenge on him in the spirit of **competition**. She has to win; she cannot lose. She has to prove she is "the best." A psoric boy could be jealous because he needs other people for protection, support, or comfort. A jealous sycotic boy needs others for the **attention**—and he will show off or act out—whatever it takes to attract attention and affection.

The grief response of sycosis is **exaggerated**. He may weep and wail, throwing himself on the floor. People in certain countries also may wail and strongly express their emotions. These emotional expressions must be viewed within the appropriate emotional and cultural context. If a homeopath treats a patient from a country where everybody wails during grief, this is not a symptom of the patient because it is part of the culture. But when such a symptom is not customary, it is a miasmatic symptom.

As homeopaths, we must be able to differentiate between a symptom as an expression of the vital force as opposed to an accepted cultural habit or behavior. If we mistakenly prescribe on culture, of course, we will miss the remedy.

Here is an example of one sycotic patient in grief. A patient in her 30s came home from work with her two children and saw her husband's car in the driveway. When she opened the door of the living room, she shouted, "We're here," but he didn't answer. She opened every door, until finally she opened the bedroom door and found her husband dead on the bed from a heart attack. She called for the doctor and called her parents. The corpse was taken away. All this happened at about 4:00 P.M. At 8:00 P.M. she was at home alone with her children, and she called the neighbor to ask if he could watch the children for her. She dressed herself nicely, went to a cafe in the marketplace, and ordered a pint of beer. She sat and enjoyed her beer. It is a small town, and some people saw her sitting there and phoned her parents. Her parents came and said, "What are you doing in this place? You have to be at home with your children. What will people think?" They were angry with her. She said, "I had to do it. It's the only thing I could do." Is this a normal reaction to grief? Most of us would find it strange that she felt she needed to do this. She wanted to be out among normal people having a good time, not with the sadness at home. This is a sycotic reaction to grief. Can we blame her? No, it is an expression of her being. This was a woman who often overdid.

Another woman who experienced grief had to go dancing. She danced all night, drinking beer, and then she felt better. Sycosis might switch on the radio, turn it up loud, and dance at home. This woman's need for loud music and dancing showed her sycosis.

Sycosis also can have excessive emotional swings, from feeling sad to feeling very manic. **Strong polarities** run all through the symptoms of sycosis. There can be boisterous laughter or temper tantrums. Instead of crying during sadness, sycosis might get very busy, working day and night, not thinking about the problem.

Sycotic patients may have depression, but in their depression they will **overdo**. They will go out drinking and try to have fun to get rid of the depression. They will drive fast while they are drunk. A sycotic suicide will be dramatic. He will crash his car or blow his brains out. He is not fastidious.

Another characteristic of sycosis is a particular kind of oversensitivity. Sycosis may be so strongly linked with another person that he can feel this person's vibrations. He can "sense" things happening beyond his five senses. This can happen between people who have a very strong relationship, such as between a mother and child or husband and wife. This is an excess of feeling that is beyond the normal.

Some compulsive behavior is sycotic because it involves doing the same thing again and again—overdoing. As always, however, we must consider why the organism is expressing a particular symptom.

Why would one need to be compulsive in his behavior? Repetition can give one security, which is psoric. For example, a patient may say, "I have to touch a certain thing several times, because if I do not, I will be ill or have bad luck, or something will happen to my family." This is psora. If the behavior is done to cut oneself off from doing better things or because of suspiciousness, in the sense of not trusting themselves, it is syphilitic. For someone who says, "Every time I come home, I have to check the door over and over to be sure that it is locked," this mistrust in oneself is syphilitic. If the compulsive behavior is excess activity, energetic overdoing, the behavior is sycotic. All can be considered ritualistic, but each behavior is performed for a different reason, from a different need, which can be understood miasmatically.

General and Physical Symptoms and Modalities of the Sycotic Miasm

Excess—overgrowth—overabundance
Sudden onset
Rapid progressions
Ameliorated by motion
Ameliorated twilight to dawn
Aggravated by dampness
Aggravated by extremes of temperature
Likes strong tastes
Desires sour, spice, salt
Likes ice
Has large features
High fevers
Enlargements/hypertrophies
Genital/urinary problems
Fishy or musty smell
Old cheese smell
Spasms
Paroxysms
Brown skin spots
Green/yellow discharges
Abdominal sleep position

Sycosis is either hot or cold; he experiences **extremes** in his internal temperature. Sticking hot feet out from under the covers is sycotic and is a typical *Medorrhinum* symptom. Sycosis may be better with cold applications.

Psora does not like the wind or a draft, but the **wind excites** and stimulates sycosis. Sycosis responds very strongly to wet and cold, being worse when damp or when in **damp places**. Sycosis may love the ocean because she feels much better there; however, we can use this kind of modality only when it is very strong.

Sycosis has **difficulty in the morning**; as the day goes on she feels better and better, until almost dawn. Her energy is better beginning at twilight and at night. Her pain is **better from movement**. If one has to jump around during his pain, say with his headache, this is a sycotic headache.

Sycosis likes **strong** food. He likes spicy tastes, red meat, salt, fat, ice cream, and sour things—sour apples, sour oranges, and lemons. He likes ice and can feel better from drinking cold beverages. He can eat fast and eat a lot. Sycosis may have a musty or fishy taste in the mouth.

In meeting a sycotic patient for the first time, we can often immediately recognize the sycotic miasm. Sycosis may have a **large** nose, one that cannot be missed. A sycotic face has a broad palate and **fleshy** red lips. Sycotic hands and feet are big, and sycotic bodies are strong and energetic. They have an abundance of hair, but the hair can fall out quite **suddenly** in circular patches, on the head or in the beard. The sycotic tongue is red. Her dental work will show fillings in the sides of the teeth, just above the gum.

The illnesses of sycosis **develop quickly**, with rapid and strong manifestations. There will be inflammations and fevers that are **fast and high**. Even in the fever, sycosis wants to move. In delirium, she will strike out. There are ruptures and discharges with thick, **greenish-yellow** pus that comes out with a lot of power—discharges from the ear, nose, and sexual organs. The discharges may have a fishy smell or a smell like old cheese. Vomit and stool may be green. Sycosis feels **better from discharges**. In general, sycosis has excessive catarrh from all mucosae.

A sycotic lung infection has a **sudden onset** with high fever, greenish-yellow sputum, and a lot of coughing that is worse in wet weather, with the sound of rattling mucus. His asthma comes on suddenly, is worse with dampness, and has copious mucus that cannot be brought up. This patient **has to move around**.

The sycotic ear infection is sudden, with **bright red** inflammation and a high fever, and the eardrum bursts. When it bursts, it discharges, and mostly this is not a big problem; the ear should drain. The sycotic child with an ear infection will have strong crying tantrums. The ear discharge comes soon after the first crying, is yellow-green and profuse, and smells like fish or old cheese.

Sycotic appendicitis is **sudden**, with a lot of pain. It must be treated quickly. When a sycotic patient comes to our practice with acute appendicitis, we do not have much time to look into her file or into the repertory. We give her the prominent remedy quickly and send her to the hospital. Perhaps even before she gets to the emergency room, the remedy will have handled the acute inflammation. Such is the rapid response of the vital force of sycosis.

The sycotic miasm shows **enlargement**, **swelling**, and suppuration. Swelling is a big part of this miasm—too much water, too much mucus, too much pus. The glands swell, and the muscles thicken or swell. Sycosis tends to have **spasmodic**, **paroxysmal** pain in his muscles. He can have **stiffness**, soreness, and lameness and is better from movement.

Brown spots on the skin are a sign of sycosis. This includes all **brown discoloration**, including freckles and melanoma. Too much pigment in certain areas shows the excess of sycosis. People who are dancers can have brown spots on the skin; you can recognize sycosis both in the need for movement and in skin.

The sycotic skin may be **oily**, in the sycotic way—there being too much. Sycotic nails are hardened, thickened. In women, the nails are likely to be long, strong, and brightly painted.

Psoric eruptions itch and burn and are red; they last a long time because the body is too weak to get rid of them. Psoric eruptions do not have discharges, but sycotic eruptions, such as acne with boils, discharge much greenish-yellow pus. The boils, vesicles, and other eruptions of sycosis are on top of the skin. Sycosis also has many acute infections. Sycosis gives **excess**, which comes out of the body. Psora is mostly too weak to push things out.

Because the origin of sycosis is in the **lower abdomen**, there is much suffering in the genital and urinary regions of the body. The sycotic miasm favors this area, with skin eruptions around the genitals, urinary tract infections, infections of the uterus and the fallopian tubes, ovaritis, and sterility—all due to inflammation. Males may have discharges, pustules on the penis, redness, prostatitis, or epididymitis. Sycosis has many **strong inflammations** in the lower abdomen, illnesses that are very quick and powerful. Other signs of sycosis include a lot of leucorrhoea—not the watery, milky discharge of psoric leucorrhoea, but a **yellowish** or **greenish discharge**—and the smell is like fish. Patients may say they do not like the smell, even after bathing. In the old days, people used brine—water with a lot of salt—to preserve fish. The Materia Medica calls this smell **fish brine**. Urine with a fishy smell is sycotic.

Consider the patient with symptoms of recurring prostatitis, swelling, redness of the glans penis, or painful ejaculations. He likes to stay up late at night and is active in the night but is weak in the morning. He will need a sycotic remedy. If he is cold and worse with wet weather, and suffers stiffness and fixed ideas, we might give *Thuja.*

When someone has had gonorrhea and allopathic treatment or antibiotics to suppress the gonorrhea, the gonorrheal discharge will go away, and the person will receive a deeper blow to the vital force. His response can be to establish a deeper illness such as **rheumatic** pains. When treated homeopathically, the greenish-yellow discharge from the urethra will come back. When this happens, the patient's initial reaction to the return of his gonorrheal symptom will be horrible. Unless we tell the patient to expect this return of his original symptoms and that it is not the illness that has come back but only the discharge, he will go again for allopathic treatment. Sometimes the discharge must continue for weeks or months. Let it come out, and as the discharge continues, he will feel much better. Things that are hidden by allopathic drugs will come out with homeopathy.

In sycosis there are **growths**, often on the genitals—a fig wart on the penis, mostly on the glans, or warts on the vulva. Sometimes there are warts around the anus. This is a sign that someone in the family history had sycosis—suppressed gonorrhea. Even without the parents themselves having had gonorrhea, their child can be born with fig warts on the penis, on the vulva, or around the anus. Sometimes these warts develop later, when the child is older. It is a sign of the sycotic miasm. These growths do not have to be around the genitals; crops of warts can occur anywhere on the body.

The sycotic miasm is full of warts, but not all warts are due to sycosis. Each miasm manifests warts in its own special way. The sycotic wart is the most beautiful wart. It is brown, often dark, usually enlarging, often with an irregular surface that has a **cauliflower** shape. Sycotic warts are jagged, rough, and hard. Patients hate them. They can be many different colors of brown but also pale. Round, soft, fleshy ones are psoric. Syphilitic warts grow deep into the skin.

In the sycotic miasm, **things grow quickly where things should not grow**—kidney stones, gallstones, exostosis of bone, fibroids in the uterus, tumors, and hemorrhoids. Simple **hemorrhoids** are sycotic, but if they are bleeding, they are syphilitic. **Gout** is sycotic. Sycosis can cause extra bone, extra tissue—an overabundance.

A heart attack could be psoric, sycotic, or syphilitic, and we must understand the difference. In thinking of what we know about the nature of sycosis, we can understand how the heart can suffer damage. It is the sycotic way to work too hard, train too much, and sleep too little. When sycosis becomes ill with a heart problem, it is due to excess. We must think about what is going on in the body and look at all the symptoms. **Hypertrophy** of the heart is sycotic because it is an increase in the volume of the heart tissue due to enlargement of the existing cells. **Tachycardia** is sycotic because it is an unusually rapid beating of the heart. **Thickening** of the blood is sycotic. **Rushing** of blood to the head is sycotic. High blood pressure is mostly sycotic, but it can be from all three miasms. When hypertension is due to kidney failure, it could be sycotic, because sycosis likes to attack the urinary tract. When hypertension is due to a destructive heart condition, it is syphilitic. When it is due to fear, it is probably psoric.

When the heart suffers an event because of a narrowing of the veins, the condition is psoric. When the veins are too large, this is sycotic. When tissue is built up where it does not belong, this is sycotic. But if the tissue builds up to protect brittle veins from breaking down, this is syphilitic.

We do not need to memorize lists of symptoms. We only have to think of how and why a process is happening in the body to determine the miasm.

The Sycotic Miasm in Infants and Children

Sycotic children also have tried to shoot me dead, but when they come into the consulting room with a toy gun, their **eyes are laughing**—it is a game. With syphilis, the eyes are cold. Sycotic children **make contact** with others, **talk** and act constantly, and stay **awake at night**. As soon as they are able to walk, they **climb** out of bed and go into the parents' room to talk at 2:00 A.M. They will be sleepy during the day, definitely in the morning. They like to be the center of attention and **perform** for others. They want lots of attention. They are jealous if others get more attention. A sycotic child also will be the "**little chief**," telling the parents what to do. **Tantrums** are sycotic. Sycotic children can be precocious, or immature, or both.

The sycotic child likes to **sleep on his abdomen** in the knee-chest position; sycotic adults are also better from lying on the abdomen.

Sycotic infants have **strong colic pains** and must be carried about. They are better from movement, from being **bounced**, from action. Sycotic infants may have a bright red rash around the anus or warts around the genital area or anus.

Their teething is **fast**, and their illnesses come on quickly, mostly in the night. They may have nightly aggravation of ear infections, with yellow-green, fishy-smelling discharges and loud crying. We know that it is sycotic **when the aggravation at night involves sycotic modalities.**

If a mother is sycotic (or if the baby is sycotic) during her pregnancy, she might be very outgoing, needing to be **busy all the time**, and have a high sex drive. The unborn baby will be active, moving and shifting as if he is perhaps playing. The mother might not be able to sleep because of the movement of the baby, especially at night, because her sycotic baby has more energy at night.

Sycotic Remedies

Kent's Repertory: **GENERALITIES; SYCOSIS;** (52): **Arg.**, **Arg-n.**, **Kali-s.**, **Med.**, **Nat-s.**, **Nit-ac.**, **Sep.**, **Staph.**, **Thuj.**, *agar.*, *apis*, *aster.*, *aur-m.*, *bar-c.*, *calc.*, *caust.*, *dulc.*, *ferr.*, *fl-ac.*, *graph.*, *iod.*, *lach.*, *lyc.*, *mang.*, *mez.*, *phyt.*, *sars.*, *sec.*, *sel.*, *sil.*, *sulph.*, alum., alumn., anac., ant-c., ant-t., aran., aur., bry., carb-an., carb-v., carbn-s., cham., cinnb., con., euphr., hep., kali-c., merc., petr., puls., sabin.

Again, the Repertory is the place to begin to learn the remedies of sycosis. For example, begin with *Argentum, Staphysagria,* or *Kali sulphuricum,* three of the nine bold remedies in *Kent's Repertory.* List the characteristic symptoms of each remedy. Decide to which miasm each symptom in the remedy belongs, then weight the remedy as to prominence of psora, sycosis, or syphilis by the number of symptoms for each miasm. Some remedies in this rubric are more sycotic than others. Knowing the prominence of each miasm in each remedy helps us give the remedy that best matches the totality of the case, including the patient's miasmatic influence.

Thuja is a strongly sycotic remedy. *Medorrhinum* is the nosode of the sycotic miasm. Some of the sycotic symptoms of *Medorrhinum* are:

- Hurried; time passes too slowly
- Extremes

- Wildness, passion, intensity
- Contrasting extremes or extremes of polarity in one person
- Feels most matters sensitively before they occur
- Loves nightlife
- Worse mornings and during the daytime, better evening or night
- Better by the sea
- Chronic or recurrent infections of pelvic organs
- Fishy odor of discharges
- Heat and swellings, especially in lower limbs
- Excrescences, condylomata
- Diarrhea after suppressed gonorrhea
- Inflammation of ovaries after suppressed gonorrhea
- Swelling of knee/rheumatic leg pains after gonorrhea

Sycosis Case 1: Man With Nephrotic Syndrome

Video Presentation and Case Description

The following discussion was captured as it occurred during a lecture, with brief video presentation and case description by Henny Heudens. Student questions and comments are italicized and appear within brackets.

A very pale man presented to me with nephrotic syndrome—a very deep illness, deeper even than asthma, which takes a long time to cure. The family health history includes diabetes, cancer of pancreas, psoriasis, and Parkinson's disease, indicating many miasmatic problems in the family.

This man is in his early 20s, with very blue, innocent eyes. He gives me the impression of being a boy. He was very clever as a child. He started school one year early, which is exceptional in his country. When he was between 5 and 8 years old, he had eczema on his back, behind his ears, and on his arms. Ointments took it away. From 6 to 10 years of age, he wept a lot when other children in school teased him about being younger. At age 17, he got mononucleosis (one-and-a-half years before the kidney problems started). From age 15 to 19, he started to gamble and became addicted to it. I learned in the second consultation that he was still a gambling addict—he had avoided telling me about this gambling problem during the initial consultation. At 18 years of age, he started to use hashish.

When he was telling me about his kidney problems, he described that he had been swimming in a lake. After swimming, he discovered that many individuals who swam in that lake developed kidney problems. He began searching the Internet to find other people who swam in the same lake that summer, wanting to find out how many others developed nephrotic syndrome so they could fight against the government or the companies who dumped waste in the lake. What does this mean? [*He is having reactions that are idealistic. Revengeful. He has energy to do this.*] Yes, but there is nothing else he can do because of his fatigue. He takes cortisone, an allopathic drug, for his kidneys, and he has to rest for hours during the day. He does not work because of his illness. Who are the fighters? [*Causticum.*] You are looking for a remedy. When you think of a remedy in the first five minutes of an interview, you will fall asleep. Try to get the history and not think of a remedy. Otherwise, you will just interview to confirm your suspicions.

So, who are the fighters? Sycotics are the fighters. What are syphilitics like in this situation? The syphilitic population generally seeks revenge. These are the people who take everything inside until they can find an outlet, which then could be violent. If this person were in a *Sulphur* state and swimming in the lake, what would happen in his mind? He might not do anything, but he would think and plan about everything he needed to read about it. He would research it. This man is very tired, but all the energy he has he spends in fighting. That means he belongs to sycosis, the fighting miasm.

He told me he had already been under homeopathic treatment two years before, and he did not like it. The other homeopath had asked him a lot of questions about things the patient did not find important, and she did not go into the origin of the case. When I asked him what he found on the Internet, he was very interested in telling me. He told me that he collected all the bits and pieces of information he had found to make a manuscript of what had happened. He said, "I will put it together and send it to the government of my country. I will ask them, how can you do such a thing—put all your dirt in the lake and let people pay for their holiday to be in a dirty lake?"

Other symptoms of this patient are swollen ankles and legs, with swelling up into his upper legs. It started when he began to gamble. He was very afraid his parents would find out that he was gambling. He also feared the banks that had given him money for his education. He lost everything, even the inheritance he would get from his parents. He could not stop gambling. Sometimes people win a little, and this makes them gamble more. Who stops gambling? Psora, because when she has enough she does not want to risk losing what she has. What does sycosis do when he wins at gambling? He wants more and more and needs the excitement that gambling gives him. From the time this patient started gambling, whenever the phone rang, he would start trembling, thinking it was his parents or the bank. He had so many debts that he thought the bank might send someone to repossess his house. He was afraid they would take everything. He was studying at the time, and he started to become very tired. About every six to eight weeks, he had to lie down and stay in his bed for a week. He felt the weakness in his shoulders and chest.

This patient gets a lot of colds; he has had one now for four months. At the end of the day, he has difficulty breathing. He loves to live in town. It is exciting—people, noise, sounds, smells. We know this belongs to the sycotic miasm. Sycotics love the activity of living in towns or cities. Syphilitics like isolation. They want to be away from everybody. What does psora like? [*Neighborhoods for protection. Close to the grocery store.*] Yes, but our sycotic remedies like the excitement of a town and nightlife. They prefer to sleep during the day.

He loves to eat French cheeses, sauces, fat, and oily food. He does not like spinach. His thirst is changeable. His sleep is good, and since he has been ill, he sleeps much better. Before becoming ill, he had very restless sleep. "Until I was 12 years old, I often rolled out of the bed onto the floor due to restlessness." His feet are hot. He likes to stick his feet out of the bed. He never wears shoes or socks inside the house. He loves company. He has an aversion to sophisticated language. He hates it, and he would like to fight with people who use it to show them that they are just normal human beings, not that educated or elevated. He has an aversion to injustice. He is writing another book about environmental problems in his country.

Fears? He has an awful fear of fire, and fear that his friends will leave him. Until the age of 12, he had an awful fear of thunderstorms and lightning. He is very impatient, and he is lazy when he is alone. He says, "I need the fun other people give me. When I am alone, I am lazy. I like change and the excitement of other surroundings. I do not like boring things in life." He had a lot of anticipation, even when he was quite well, about going to university. When he had to take a test, he was very anxious about performing well. Now he has stopped studying because of his weakness.

Are you thinking about his aversion to injustice? Are you thinking again of *Causticum*? Who of you here have no aversion to injustice? When is this reaction extreme? If you tell a lie about me, do I like it? No, but if I am psora, how will I react? [*Worrying about what people think about me.*] Yes, psora would suffer inside, because the more fuss one makes, the more people gossip. If I am syphilitic and you tell a lie about me, I will wait for my chance to get you for it and brood about it until I can act. If I am sycotic, I will react right on the spot; I will react immediately.

To react when somebody does an injustice to you is not in itself a symptom. But when someone tells you he hates his father because of something that happened when he was three years old, this means he cannot forgive or that he "dwells on past disagreeable occurrences." When is a reaction to an injustice a symptom? [*When it is all the person can think about.*] Yes, when they turn their lives around to deal with it.

Recently, sexual crimes have been occurring in Belgium. One of the parents whose child was killed has been on television every day and has gathered 250,000 people together in the capital to march against child abuse. We all know he cannot get his child back. I think it is a healthy reaction to overcome his grief, but why is he doing this? He cannot save his own child; it is to save other children. We all know people who start causes after an injustice has been done to them. This is an extreme reaction.

Why does our patient have his cause? To get more money for his gambling. He is looking for other people to support his fight. It is totally selfish. The way he reacts shows his inner personality. What kind of miasm do we see in his symptoms? Is this clearly sycosis? Show me the signs and symptoms. [*Excessive gambling, loves nightlife and excitement, likes change, likes company, swelling, has fear of being found out.*] Sycosis likes to hide how bad he is, but fear of being found out could be psora also. [*He is impatient, and he is slim, with those wonderful, blue innocent eyes.*] Does this look like sycosis? [*He could be tubercular because of the shape of his body—wasted, no energy, and needing "kicks," collapsing at an early age.*]

Sycosis Case 1—Analysis

This patient is a man with a possibly tubercular shape but who loves sycotic things. Also, he likes to swim. What must we do in such a case? [*Take the rest of the case.*] His former homeopath gave him *Phosphorus*—for a wonderful, sweet, boy. There are *Phosphorus* characteristics in this man, for example, fear of thunderstorms until he was 12 years old, very social, outgoing. So how do we discern the correct remedy for this person? The two possibilities so far are *Phosphorus* and *Causticum*, a tubercular remedy and a sycotic remedy, respectively. This man is very ill at every level. Look at the timeline. When did he acquire the gambling problem? One-and-a-half years before mononucleosis, about the same time as the kidney problems. His health was quite good until he was 12, but his eczema was suppressed by ointment, and then he became quite ill.

What was his background? All miasms are in the family. He is a deeply ill man. When you list the symptoms—fear of fire, fear of thunderstorms, anticipation, needs company, likes gambling—which miasms remain? Sycotic and tubercular. There are many similarities to both in his history.

My way of choosing in such a case—where two miasms or two remedies are running the same course for the mental and emotional symptoms—is quite easy. I note the pathology the patient has developed. If he really were tubercular, what pathology would he develop? Lung problems. If he were sycotic, what pathology would he develop? Genital, urinary, or abdominal problems.

He is a bit out of breath at the end of the day. This could be tubercular, but if he were strongly tubercular, what would he get after the suppression of his eczema? [*Asthma.*] Yes, perhaps asthma. What is happening now with his kidney disease? The weakness is going on; he is becoming more and more ill. What kind of remedy is the most appropriate, or which miasm is most prominent at this moment? [*Sycosis.*] When I first saw the patient, I too thought of a tubercular remedy. How might a sycotic person look? Bull-like, muscular, compact, solid. He does not present this way. After a sycotic remedy, you probably will see another layer. Do we agree that he needs a sycotic remedy? Now we look at which sycotic remedy he needs.

[*Medorrhinum.*] This is a definite possibility. Another possibility? [*Thuja.*] [*Staphysagria.*] [*Lycopodium.*] Let's reason now. Why *Lycopodium*? [*It has all three miasms.*] What's another thing for *Lycopodium*? [*Kidneys.*] [*Cowardly, not wanting to confront his parents.*] Does the following scenario show cowardice? Let's say you're a gambler and that all your bank savings, even your possessions, are gone, and you have sold your future inheritance. No one would want to admit this. I do not think he is a coward; his reaction is quite normal. [*We have anticipation, gambling.*]

We go on to *Staphysagria.* [*The idea of writing a book and being very sensitive and very sweet, may have problems with kidneys. Staphysagria can be wild or very sweet.*] This man seems quite soft and sweet, not wild. Anything else for *Staphysagria?* [*Sensitive to what the family will say.*] If I went to Las Vegas next week and lost all of my money, how would I feel when I have to fly home and tell my husband? This would be difficult for anyone, so not a good symptom.

Thuja is definitely sycotic. Who's in favor of this? [*He is secretive, does not fit in, has suppression.*] All four remedies have suppression though. What else? [*Weakness.*] He is weak. [*Thuja is strongly sycotic and tubercular.*] No, *Thuja* is not very strongly tubercular. How does *Thuja* usually behave? [*Puts up a front; hides, unable to talk about personal problems.*] Yes, but this man was very open with me. He loves company and excitement. This does not belong to *Thuja,* who is mostly withdrawn, with things on his mind but not showing it. You have to see how somebody comes into the consulting room. Why does he come? He says he has two problems: nephrotic syndrome and "I am a gambler." We all know some patients who come because they have a problem with the toenail on their right foot. During the consultation, you may discover that the real problem is something like impotency. Openness does not belong to *Thuja.* What is usually the case when people haven't enough energy? Usually, they are chilly. What is *Thuja* sensitive to? [*Cold or wet.*] I will not tell you that they won't ever swim in a lake because it is too cold, but mostly they do not like to be exposed to wet, cold things.

What indicates *Medorrhinum* as a possible remedy for him? [*It is a kidney remedy, loves nightlife, gambling, excitement, salt, fat.*] The salt and fat desire of *Medorrhinum* is equal to that of *Sulphur.* When we consider *Medorrhinum,* what symptoms do we see in him? [*Anticipation.*] Yes; do not forget that *Medorrhinum* has anticipation in the remedy. What else is a characteristic? [*Hot feet, extremism, likes bare feet.*] [*Green discharges, which he does not have.*] [*Likes seaside, likes sour, is social.*]

Taking all these symptoms up to now into consideration, what speaks for or against *Sulphur* for this patient? We know that *Sulphur* likes salt, sour, extremism, and nightlife.

[*There is not the theorizing of Sulphur here.*] Yes, that's right; this man takes action and does not just theorize. He is writing a book with what little energy he has.

[*Sulphur works in the mind more than Medorrhinum.*] Yes, but *Sulphur* also can have strong physical symptoms.

If we compare *Medorrhinum* symptoms with those of *Sulphur*, we have another problem. *Sulphur* is mostly psoric. *Medorrhinum* is more focused in the genitals and urinary tract. Why? Because it is inherited sycosis. To prescribe for him and make a differentiation between *Medorrhinum* and *Sulphur*, where is the decision? [*Background, history.*] The miasmatic history is important. His family background is one of sycosis and syphilis—a mixed case. We could start with psora, except that we have gambling and nephrotic syndrome. Before, there was eczema, but that is gone. What could his miasm be for just the eczema? Maybe psora. So, when the eczema was suppressed, what did he get? Gambling addiction. You will see this only when there is a sycotic background. What did the suppression do to the organism? He was healthier when the psora was expressing itself on the skin. Once that outlet was suppressed or blocked, his organism shifted the disturbance to active sycosis.

> *When something suppresses the organism, something else from the internal illness will come out. The symptom may be suppressed, but the illness goes on and needs expression, and the illness will refocus and produce symptoms in another part of the organism.*

His suppressed eczema went into a deep mental problem. If we give him a psoric remedy now, what will happen? [*The best thing would be for nothing to happen.*] His organism is asking for a sycotic remedy. If his nephrotic syndrome were suppressed with cortisone, what might be the result? The syphilitic problems would emerge, then deep depression would be a possibility. This would be quite logical in his situation—very ill at a young age, losing all his money—so depression could be the next step. This is what we see in practice. Happily, he comes now while we see his sycosis. What will happen if we give him a sycotic remedy? His sycosis will become inactive, and his psora will become active. He might develop breathing problems because the tubercular influence is in him. The cancer miasm is in him. When a disturbance is in you, what has to happen? [*It has to come out.*]

When he is back to psora, how will he be? [*Healthier.*] It means that if the syphilis comes out after this, it will come out in a very mild way, not destroying the body. Subsequent syphilitic expressions will be more superficial in nature, possibly with a skin irritation or a throat infection. I prescribed a sycotic remedy. He needed *Medorrhinum.*

[*Isn't nephrotic syndrome syphilitic because it affects a deep organ?*] Nephrotic syndrome can be due to a combination of miasms, almost as deep as cancer. It is very difficult to treat. It is hard work because there is real destruction in the kidneys. Sometimes we can only stop the destruction. However, in some cases, we can repair destructive damage. I remember two cases of young girls in their teens who came to me because of backaches. Both girls did a lot of sports. We stopped their sports during the treatment because we had the impression that they had overdone and that the sports caused the backache. When they did not improve on the first remedy, we sent them for x-rays. Both girls showed an infection in the vertebrae, and a piece of vertebra was lost from the infection. What miasm do you have here? [*Syphilis.*] Yes, infection that eats the bone. The remedy was changed, and the sports were stopped again. I asked for another x-ray, which showed that the vertebrae were totally repaired. How is this possible? We can see this deep level of healing after we successfully treat the patients' miasmatic illnesses. These girls were still young enough that bone growth and bone repair were possible for them. They were strong, and had a lot of energy for healing. It was wonderful to see how the body could repair itself.

Sycosis Case 1—Followups

Let's follow what happened with this man. He asked if he could stop his drugs, but I told him to wait until he felt better and then to gradually decrease them over several months. I also asked him to contact me when he felt better. I did not see him until 15 months later. His energy was much better; he gradually eliminated the cortisone (the allopathic drug for the kidneys) and started to work in an office. He could only work 50 percent of the time because he was tired after half a day; his ankles started to swell again. What's going on with him? [*Energy is much better, started to work, to pay his debt.*] He stopped gambling. He said it was difficult for him not to gamble, but he felt he had to stop; yet, last month his fear about his parents came back, even without gambling. He started getting anxious again. He relapsed, even without gambling, but in a very mild way—on both the physical and emotional levels. His kidney disease is a severe illness, and he is in an obvious relapse. Does he need a remedy? Yes—a repetition of *Medorrhinum* in the same potency (200C).

He called me two years later for another consultation, saying he felt bad, even worse than before. He could not work anymore and had stopped writing. He had gone to his parents to tell them, "Not only are my kidneys better, but also I stopped the gambling, and I work a whole day now to pay back all of the inheritance." This was a good exchange of feelings between his father and him and shows that he now felt that he could tell his parents about the gambling. However, his father reacted negatively and said, "You are just like your uncle, who did the same thing. It would be better to drown yourself than to tell me these things." Then the patient started to have sleepless nights because of thinking about all that he'd done wrong. He again started to have kidney symptoms and swelling of his ankles.

I asked him about his reaction to his father. Why? [*You wanted to know whether he was still sycotic.*] If he cannot sleep because of guilt, it is a psoric symptom. Yes, I wanted to know if he needed *Medorrhinum* again or some other remedy. Is he still sycotic? The inability to sleep due to guilt is a strong psoric symptom. If he were sycotic, he might have been angry, yelling and telling his father that he was unjust. Instead, the patient said he was totally blocked, speechless. "I couldn't react, and I had the feeling I had to cry, but I couldn't. I feel so sad that my father didn't understand why I told the things I did." This is psora coming. When I asked him how he felt, he said, "Weak and sad. If I go on this way, I will have to stop working again. I feel so weak I cannot perform."

The expression of psora is not totally present, only the feeling of it. Sleeplessness can be found in any miasm. If he is sleepless from excitement, it is sycosis. If he is not sleeping because of revengeful feelings, it is syphilis.

His ankles are swelling again. If he does not get a homeopathic remedy, he will go on cortisone. We have to do something. [*Psorinum has swelling of the ankles and sleeplessness day and night.*]

He has sleeplessness because of the guilt; nothing else has changed. My reasoning is this: He is much healthier than before on the mental level. Now he has guilt and some new emotions. His disease shows the same way. If he were really in a psoric state, he would have more psoric symptoms—perhaps itching with no eruption because the body was too weak to produce it. I think we have a healthier *Medorrhinum* than before but still *Medorrhinum*.

I repeated the remedy, even when some psoric symptoms were coming. Should I have waited before prescribing again? [*No.*] I had to do something. If we were to prescribe a psoric remedy, what could the remedy do? Either suppress or push his sycosis into a stronger, more active state. It is correct to give a different remedy when the total picture changes, but this is the same picture, only healthier.

I saw this patient again one-and-a-half years later. He phoned to request an appointment as soon as possible. This was the first time he had ever done this. Even with his deeper disease, he had never asked for an urgent appointment. He had a big skin eruption that itched a lot. "Now that I feel good about going out to meet people, look how I am. I met a nice girl."

There is itching and eruption. Now we have the expression of psora. What should we do? [*Take the case.*] Yes, even more carefully than before, so we do not suppress him and push him back to where he was. I took his case, and I told him I could not do anything at that moment. He was not happy with me, but I knew that we had to wait. I knew his skin eruption would not go away in two or three weeks. I asked him to wait a month or a few weeks to see whether his case could develop in such a way that I could prescribe a remedy.

At a moment when there are almost no modalities and no other picture, keep your hands off! You have to be sure when you give a remedy.

I asked him to write down any other later changes in feeling, eating, or drinking and said he could phone me when he had more information. He worked half-days and went to university the other half-days. He had resumed his studies and was working to pay back the debts. He was studying to make a good future. He told me that some evenings when he was alone in the house and no friends were phoning him, he still had the urge sometimes to go out to gamble. He could control it, but he asked me how long it would take until he could get rid of this idea. "Do I have to wait until I'm 80 years old?" This is why I wanted to wait. He was in a healthier state, but *Medorrhinum* still showed itself, even though weaker or softer. If I gave him another dose of *Medorrhinum,* it might stop the eruption and force the illness deeper.

I told him not to wait six months but to phone me in one month. I wanted to keep him in homeopathic treatment. If he were to be out of contact with me, the cortisone cream would be easy to take. During his last phone call, he said that his eczema was much better; it was only on the legs now. It has taken seven months for the eczema to improve. His kidneys are better, and he is studying and working.

It is always our lesson to respect the vital force. The vital force works with homeopathy on its own schedule.

We cannot interfere, even if it takes two years before his eczema is gone. We are often tempted to overdo. One of our problems is not being able to wait when people ask for help. We all have an allopathic education, which means that when a patient pays for a consultation, we feel badly when we cannot do anything. Most of the time, if they are on the correct remedy and you prescribe again, it is the wrong thing to do. Even though we know that we should prescribe only when necessary, it is sometimes difficult to know when it is necessary and when to keep our hands off.

We have a history of cancer, syphilis, and the tubercular state. What do we do with this? We wait. Sometime he will see his father again, and his body will express what it needs.

Homeopaths must deal with an inner struggle between what we know we must do as homeopaths and what we emotionally want to do for the patient. It is good to have compassion, but we must not lose our objectivity. Objectivity is our first weapon for cure. We must know the rules of our profession.

Sycosis Case 2: Boy With Recurrent Throat Infections

Video Presentation and Case Description

The following discussion was captured as it occurred during a video presentation and case description by Henny Heudens. Student questions and com-

ments appear within brackets. In the interview portions, "HH" indicates a question or comment by Henny, and "P" indicates the patient.

HH—What do you like to do in your free time?"
P—Dance.
HH— For how long?
Father—Since he was four years of age.

This 11-year-old boy has dark brown hair, is very handsome and refined, and loves to dance. Of course, you never give a remedy because somebody dances. Listen to his voice for a while, and then we'll turn off the sound and only watch the child and I will tell you the case. He is a happy child. At home, he behaves openly, but at school he is withdrawn and silent. He works well in school and has a good temperament.

He has had problems since he had a Bacillus Calmette-Guerin (BCG) vaccine at two years of age. He looks tubercular, giving a similar physical impression as in the sycotic man in the case we just finished. This boy's problem is recurrent throat infections that started when he was two years old—after vaccination against tuberculosis. He was apathetic for two weeks after the vaccination, with swollen tonsils and swelling in all the glands in his neck. He was very weak for the two weeks of the apathetic period and remained weak for an additional two weeks. Tonsillitis started again, with the same pattern of weakness afterward. This pattern repeated itself again and again. He began homeopathic treatment at seven years of age and has had several remedies:

- *Pulsatilla* with no result.
- *Carcinosin* helped him a little, but the second dose of *Carcinosin* had no result. Other potencies produced no reaction.
- *Silica* with no result, repeated several times.
- *Tuberculinum* with no result.

The mother had gonorrhea nine years before the birth of the child. During the pregnancy, the mother had nausea for four weeks, loss of blood, was very excited during the pregnancy, and could not sleep. If you could see the mother, you would see she that is very worn out.

The child had five teeth at birth! Until four months of age, he had much colic, with screaming. Before the vaccination, even when he had a high fever, he felt fine. His parents could not believe he had a fever by how he behaved; yet his fevers were very high. With each recurrence of tonsillitis, he became weaker. When he was four years of age, the family adopted another boy. The patient did not seem to be jealous; he felt fine to have a little brother. His behavior with his brother was good. Until age six years, he had a lot of aphthae in the mouth, loose stools, and itching on the penis. His hobby has been dancing since he was four years old. He dances now and wants to dance professionally when he grows up or do something involved with art.

In school he is quiet but is very expressive at home. When he is at home, the house is alive. With some children, you may feel like there is a storm or a wind in your house. This is the feeling the parents have. When he was two-and-a-half years old, he went on holiday with his grandmother, whom he loves very much. After he came home, he did not want to go anywhere without his mother. Since then, he clings to his mother. He has a fear that someone will take him or abuse him; even since he was very small and did not know what abuse was, he has had a fear of men who could do harm to him.

He has fear of injections. He loves animals. When his little brother has a small accident, he will calm him down. When an animal has something wrong with it, he cannot be consoled. He totally cares for them and worries about them very much. At home, there is a pet rabbit in a cage in the kitchen; as soon as the boy comes home, he takes the rabbit out of the cage. He walks with him in the village and explains everything to him. He buys toys for the rabbit. He is very proud of the rabbit, how the rabbit plays, how he can dance. The boy is very warm at night and has to stick his feet out; he never sleeps totally under the covers. He prefers quite healthy food, not too sweet, and likes his vegetables with sour sauces. He has aversion to spinach and to cauliflower, and he does not like meat very much. He craves ice cream and hot rice porridge, which is quite soft and made with a little sugar. (Most children in Belgium adore it.)

He talks very fast, and his behavior toward his brother is like that of a mother or teacher. He likes to teach all the time; he even teaches the rabbit. When he has pain in his throat, his glands are very swollen. He is patient and weak when ill. His appetite is totally normal when he has a fever. His fever is worse in the morning than in the evening. When he has fever, he does not drink a lot. He likes coffee for his tonsillitis. He has crusts on alternating sides of his nose. He likes warm drinks, except with fever. He normally likes orange juice. He sleeps on his right side.

What are the indications for the remedy he needs? I am sure you have heard symptoms that do not belong to the remedy that seems most similar. Many cases can look like several remedies. This is a problem in homeopathy. He looks like a tubercular child and has had problems since his BCG vaccination, and yet I did not give him *Tuberculinum* or another tubercular remedy. One of the strong points in this case is that the mother had gonorrhea; yet this by itself does not mean he needs that nosode. What are his characteristic symptoms on which to prescribe? We have:

- Heat
- Green crusts in the nose
- Born with five teeth (excessive)
- High fever, without symptoms of illness or pain (This can also be *Syphilinum* or *Tuberculinum.*)
- History of gonorrhea in mother
- Swelling of glands (right after the vaccination) (This could be tubercular or sycotic.)
- Desire for orange juice
- Talks very fast
- Very attractive, wears bright clothes (His mother always dresses in dark colors.)
- Desires sour
- Love for animals—extreme
- Genital itching at age six years (*Sulphur* can also have genital redness and itching.)
- Aphthae—mouth

Some illnesses are due to predisposition. In our neighborhood, I see some children at three and four years of age playing in the mud, and they may even eat the mud but are never ill. Some children who are bathed twice a day are often more ill. Of course, I do not tell people not to bathe their children, but their susceptibility to certain conditions may determine whether they become ill from them.

How many people think there is a draft in here? Why do some people feel a draft and others do not feel it? Does someone *feel* a draft of air, or is there *really* a draft of air? For those in front of the windows, there is a draft of air. If the people not sitting in front of the windows feel a draft, this is a symptom. Those who get sick after exposure to drafts of air are those who are very sensitive to drafts of air. Some people are more susceptible to getting sick after getting wet. Some will get a bladder infection from wearing wet clothes. This is because of their susceptibility. Some little girls get vaginal infections because they put something in their vaginas or because they do not wipe properly, while others who have the same behavior do not suffer illness from it. Those who get the infections are those who are susceptible.

What else is unusual for this boy? [*The sense that someone would attack him or come after him.*] Yes, he does not want to leave the parents anymore. We also have:

- Fear of men, of being pursued
- Power, his "alive" personality
- Dancing
- Fever, better evening
- Hot feet

His remedy is *Medorrhinum.* [*He can be very outgoing at home and quiet at school.*] Yes, this belongs to the remedy—remember the polarity. How is his dancing expressed? He has been dancing for seven years and wants to be a professional dancer. This is more than the usual desire of children to dance occasionally. This expresses his desire to move. You do not have to have a jumpy, shouting personality to need *Medorrhinum.* Dancing could also be tubercular. Sticking his hot feet out of the covers is sycotic and is a typical *Medorrhinum* symptom. Tubercular patients don't do this because they are cold.

Love of animals can be seen in both the sycotic and tubercular miasms. Also swollen glands. Excessive growth of teeth can be precocity since they came in so early. Dancing is the sycotic desire for movement. His shape is tubercular more than sycotic. His cough is much more tubercular. How is a tubercular fever? It is mostly remittent and usually low-grade, not a high fever. Tubercular fevers usually come at nighttime. He gets his fevers in the morning, and he is better in the evening. This is a sycotic symptom.

You might think he has a tubercular presentation—skinny, long shiny hair, refined. However, with regard to his symptoms, which of you would prescribe a tubercular remedy? Miasmatically, the symptoms are sycotic. Where did he get his illness? His susceptibility is due to the suppressed gonorrhea of his mother. What brought out his symptoms? The vaccinations; however, thinking that he is tubercular simply because he was vaccinated with a tubercular substance is isopathic thinking and incorrect to his treatment. He reacted after vaccinations because he was already sycotic and he needs a sycotic remedy.

A tubercular remedy would cover only part of the patient. The best remedy we can give now is the sycotic one that covers the whole patient. This is an example of someone who has been given many remedies, but they were all given on a piece of the picture, not on the totality of symptoms. We can do this with well-known remedies and with less well-known remedies. When taking a case, we should make a list of the symptoms and analyze the miasm of each symptom. I do not believe in voices from heaven that tell us, "This is a *Medorrhinum* patient." Homeopathy is hard work, but when we understand the case miasmatically, we have a much easier time knowing what is needed. I gave him *Medorrhinum* 200C.

Sycosis Case 2—Followup

One year later, the boy's mother described his reaction to the remedy. The day after *Medorrhinum* 200C, the boy needed to urinate 8 to 10 times the first night. Two days later, he was very excited; they could not stop him from talking. Nine days after the remedy, he got diarrhea that lasted for two days. Two months after the remedy, he got a cold. This is a wonderful reaction, a good discharge. Why the excitement two days after the remedy? [*Another discharge.*] Diarrhea was another discharge. He had a yellow discharge from the penis that lasted several weeks. He now feels fine. The symptoms are gone, and he feels in harmony. His mother wishes he had gotten the remedy at four years of age. I have patients who are 89 and 92 years old who are doing well with homeopathy. I have to look at their birth dates because I cannot believe how old they are.

When you treat children, you are protecting the next generation because when they will marry, they will have children who will be healthier.

Allopathic doctors can treat people and make them feel better. We tend to see the people who are *not* helped by allopathy, but allopaths are able to help many people. I never want allopathic treatment for myself if I can get help with homeopathy, and I have never needed allopathy. However, there are patients who take antibiotics once and feel fine. Some have taken sleeping pills, and they were not suppressed. Homeopaths often see the more sensitive patients—often those who *do* react badly to allopathy.

The first consultation requires a lot of focus, and when I do the first consultation very well, I truly understand the case and the correct remedy is clear. The trouble starts when we give the wrong remedy the first time and there is a reaction. [*Must you have other positive signs that the remedy worked? I might not be sure that urination or excitement is good.*] Never stop a discharge after you know the remedy has worked. Do something only if the patient's life is in danger. If a patient with Crohn's disease or ulcerative colitis comes to you with a discharge, do you expect them to have more discharge? No, you expect to stop the diarrhea. However, patients usually can have a discharge a long time without it making them really weak.

Remedy Differentials

Let's compare *Medorrhinum* and *Sulphur* characteristics since they share similar symptoms:

Symptom	***Medorrhinum***	***Sulphur***
Discharge	Green	Yellow, offensive
Weakness	Exhaustion, weak joints	Weak back, slumps
Fever	Morning	Early morning at 11 A.M.
Desires sour	Very strong—unripe fruit	Averse sour
Love for animals	Excessive	Not in repertory
Itching genitals	Yes	Yes
Fear of men	Not in repertory	Yes
Power	High energy/whirlwind	Yes, but less so
Outgoing/social ability	Yes	Yes
Dancing	Yes—movement	Not so much
Hot feet	Yes—cold toes	Yes

There is much similarity between *Sulphur* and *Aurum* and between *Aurum* and *Medorrhinum*. Comparing these symptoms using computer repertories reveals how many symptoms they have in common.

How does this little boy love animals? [*Extremely*]. And he loves his animals in an active way because he can play with them, dress them up, take them for a walk, talk to them, be active with them. Does sycosis usually buy a small dog? No, he probably will buy one that is fast and quick—a real dog, not a toy. What kind of animal does psora buy? A big one for protection. Of course, all the miasms could buy a big dog. The key is to ask why they buy it. I know a family with little dogs—complete with combs, brushes, toys, shampoo, a bed, and hairdressers! What does that represent? [*Excess of sympathy.*] They treat the little dogs like toys. The rubric for this is **MIND; CHILDISH *behavior*.** The family members behave like five-year-olds, treating the dogs like dolls. If somebody keeps a big mean dog that tries to bite people who pass the house, this is syphilitic. This is illness.

Who likes plants and flowers? Almost everybody. When somebody does not like them, it is a symptom. Plants are alive, but if we try to discuss our cases with plants, what does that mean? When someone has delusions that plants can hear and speak back, giving them human qualities, that is crossing the line. There are cases of people who fell in love with plants and had conversations with plants. This is as ill as someone who hates everything that is green. Every patient presents the homeopath with a challenge to find the symptoms. This is my love for homeopathy—it is always new.

CHAPTER 4

Tuberculosis and the Tubercular Miasm

As with syphilis, there is a difference between the disease of tuberculosis and the tubercular miasm. The miasm is the result of suppressing the disease of tuberculosis in past generations, which causes past problems to continue forward and resurface in subsequent generations in various ways.

When we speak of someone "having a miasm," we mean that this person has received an energetic layer or disease pattern and, consequently, now exhibits the particular characteristic influence of the original disease. This disease pattern is established generally in three ways:

1. The patient contracted the disease.
2. The patient received the miasmatic influence from someone in the family—someone in the family's history at some time in the past contracted the actual disease for which the miasm is named.
3. The patient contracted the miasmatic influence through vaccination against the disease.

This energetic influence can set in motion one's propensity to diseases of the tubercular miasm. Maybe one develops disease or maybe not, but the marks of the diseases of one's ancestors are passed on and inherited, just as one inherits the genetic propensity for the blue or brown eyes of his ancestors. It is a pity that we call the tubercular miasm "tubercular," because it makes us think of the disease—unless we understand well the idea of miasms. When I say tubercular or tuberculosis, I will mean the miasm unless otherwise noted.

More complicated cases reveal the mixing of the miasms. Psora is in everyone. Without psora, we would be perfect, but we know humans are imperfect. When psora is there, sycosis or syphilis can come in. One person can have psora plus sycosis or psora plus syphilis, or one can have all three miasms together.

If in one patient there is psora, sycosis, and syphilis, another "miasmatic child" may be born. This "child" would be the tubercular miasm.

Having all three miasms in one organism does not ensure the tubercular miasm, but one might have it. If one has only psora and sycosis, these two alone are insufficient to bring forth the tubercular miasm. The same is true if only psora and syphilis are present—the tubercular miasm will not establish itself. Although syphilis and/or sycosis can exist one without the other, the tubercular miasm can only exist where the other three miasms are already present.

Hahnemann said that when a patient has symptoms from all three miasms, he could be certain that it was a difficult case. Today, this margin of difficulty in curing patients has been magnified even further by the existence of a fourth miasm. To truly cure a patient, we must be able to recognize the path of the disturbance and understand how to manage our patients as they wind their way through each miasm on their way to health.

When there is evidence of each miasm in one case, we must first treat the miasm whose symptoms are the most prominent, because this is where the vital force is expressing itself most strongly.

This is not easy. These cases will probably need more than one remedy to be cured. If one remedy cannot cover all the symptoms, then we have to use different remedies to treat miasms as they surface. In managing these cases, one miasm will settle down, only to have another speak up and ask for help.

We must always keep a keen eye on what needs to be cured in our patients. When these moments shift, we must understand what is happening and be ready to treat correctly.

In Hahnemann's time, the tubercular miasm was not prominent because most patients who contracted tuberculosis often died young or did not marry or produce children and, therefore, did not pass on the disease effect as a miasm. In his time, there were still patients with only psora. In our time, people with only psora are very, very rare. Most patients have two or more miasms.

When a patient is first infected with the tuberculosis bacilli, the primary effects of the disease often go unrecognized. Here is a medical description of the early process of the tuberculosis infection:

> "PRIMARY TUBERCULOSIS: When the tuberculosis bacilli first reach the lungs and begin to multiply there, the body rushes its defenses to the infected area and almost always is successful in inactivating the infection. Some of the bacteria are killed, and the rest are covered by tough scar tissue. Although the imprisoned bacilli remain alive, they are powerless. The first infection usually causes no symptoms. An adult with active tuberculosis often experiences fatigue and vague pains in the chest, which may go unnoticed, since they are often not severe enough to attract attention. The most well known symptoms of tuberculosis—cough, expectoration of purulent sputum, fever, night sweats, and hemorrhage from the lungs—do not appear in the early, most easily curable stages of the disease; often their appearance is delayed until a year or more after the initial exposure to the bacilli." (From *Encyclopedia and Dictionary of Medicine*, Benjamin Frank Miller and Claire Brackman Keane, 1972, page 987.)

Children may experience fever and weight loss. Adults may feel unexplainably tired or develop a little cough or fever. Mostly, one who is infected will not feel well for some days and then will get a little better, but may continue with some episodes of night sweats. Crowded, poor living conditions, and inadequate rest and nutrition increase the susceptibility in children and in individuals with lowered or compromised immune systems.

Tubercular patients are usually cheerful and optimistic. When you see them, their eyes are brilliant. In the past, in the Western world, patients with tuberculosis were pale, with a flush on their cheeks. They did not look very ill; in fact, they were thought beautiful because of their high color. They were lean and elegant. Because they did not have a lot of physical energy, they spent time in thought, dreamed lovely notions, had creative ideas, and did wonderfully artistic things.

In the history of the art world, many wonderful artists had active tuberculosis disease. They secluded themselves, working very hard day and night—coughing and spitting blood—to finish their work. They had an urge to create great works of art, enough to disregard their health and their need for rest. An artist often is driven by this urge to create. A tubercular artist is someone who pushes the edge, responding feverishly to each inspiration, attempting to live every moment in creative passion or celebration.

History is filled with the biographies of artists who lived intensely and passionately, focused on their art, often without enough money for good food, without a certain balance of circumstances.

A tubercular musician might work day and night on his opera, without eating or drinking, until he finishes his work. Then, he will celebrate and have fun because he has worked so hard. And then he will play just as hard as he worked, not stopping until he has to work again. There is a definite pattern. Often these people will work at night. Some artists go to work at 10:00 P.M. and work until 7:00 A.M. Then they are tired and have to drink a little. They go to bed at 11:00 A.M., sleep all day, and are awake in the evening. Tubercular musicians work and celebrate, often until late in the night. They like to travel and may drink alcohol or use other recreational drugs.

Prior to the development of antibiotics, there were no drugs with which to treat tuberculosis. Wealthy patients went to sanatoriums in Switzerland. There, in the mountains, there was an abundance of fresh clean air and the opportunity to lie down outside and breathe deeply. Good rich food was served, with lots of cream and milk for calories, to strengthen the body and help the patient gain weight against the wasting. There was no nightlife—only the moon and the stars and snow, which made for quiet and peaceful surroundings. There was physical rest. Patients were not allowed much activity until their health improved. These treatments were very wise. The disease did not go away altogether, but after one or two years spent away in the mountains, one's body could cope with the illness.

Today, this combination of rest, fresh air, and good rich food is rarely the prescribed treatment for tuberculosis. Today's medicine treats with drugs. Rather than resting, patients continue working while taking their drugs, and then they are "cured." With drugs, they can still do everything they did before they became ill. They eat their awful junk food and struggle with the stress of their work. Although these drugs are usually unable to kill all of the tubercle bacilli, they are able to suppress the active tuberculosis disease. Happily, those who have the tubercular miasm in this time are mostly those with ancestors whose tuberculosis diseases were treated with rest, fresh mountain air, and good food. In the future, we will see more children of tubercular patients whose disease has been suppressed with antitubercular drugs.

After tuberculosis had been widely spread because of poverty and poor nourishment, there came a time of better hygiene, good nourishment, and warm houses. For about 60 to 70 years, there were very few cases of active tuberculosis disease, not because of homeopathy, but because of good hygiene and better living conditions.

Now, in many countries, the disease of tuberculosis is spreading again, especially in young people with excessive hobbies. We must ask ourselves why this is happening. We have good houses and good food, plenty of air although not always of good quality, yet we see the disease flaring up again. We must consider the possibility of widespread suppression. Our ability to withstand or overpower the disease, even with improved living conditions, somehow has been altered. Has the disease increased in vitality? One possible contributing factor is a weakening of our immune systems due to the use and misuse of allopathic drugs and vaccinations. We are seeing many more respiratory infections in our clinics than ever before.

We spoke of the sycosis of those of our younger generation who are spending the weekends in all-night, all-weekend disco "raves." These places are crowded and dark. The young dance and sweat. They emerge on Sunday night exhausted, having been there all weekend with poor air, lots of smoke, no rest, much dancing and excitement, and often drug use. This is one circumstance/environment in which the disease of tuberculosis is being spread again. Some of these young people who are susceptible are getting tuberculosis, which is then suppressed with powerful drugs. What is the future for their children?

Remember that susceptibility to tuberculosis is established in a patient when there is a family history of the tuberculosis disease, when a person is tested for the disease, or when a person receives the vaccination to inoculate against the disease. When the other miasms are already present in the family and the parent is vaccinated against tuberculosis, their children receive the susceptibility. Forty years ago, children were given BCG, an anti-tuberculosis vaccine, at three days of age. When these children were not strong, they got the problems of the tubercular miasm. In an attempt to control the spread of a disease, doctors again have unknowingly created a miasm. Because of vaccinations and testing, I believe our youth are more susceptible to coughs, bronchitis, and allergies. BCG and other vaccinations create weaknesses in human beings.

Imagine that a child with tubercular ancestors is born, gets a throat infection when very young, and is given antibiotics. He was born with the inherited tendency of lung problems and has been further weakened with antibiotics. Now he can get bronchitis or pneumonia or go deeper into asthma. Because this child has the wasting possibility and the quick movement of the tubercular miasm, his vital force can be easily and severely suppressed.

Think about the prominence of allergies and asthma today. When I was a child, it was hardly known. I lived in a large town, and one neighbor had asthma. Everybody talked about his asthma because it was so unusual. It is remarkable to see how common asthma has become in so few years. Many adults and children are now dying from asthma or are suffering severe consequences from taking the drugs needed to keep their airways open. Medical suppression has decreased the health of the population. We live longer, but at what cost to our quality of life?

We are told that some children will outgrow asthma after ages 7 to 12 years. Their course of treatment includes various forms of steroids and inhalers, and if this treatment is "successful," the allergic symptoms stop. (These days, it is common to take steroids for many things.) Some children "outgrow" the allergic symptoms with drugs, but their disease grows inward rather than showing itself outward. If they are weak and there is a family history, perhaps they will develop cancer. Suppression of childhood illnesses may be why cancer is spreading in susceptible young children. Others go through their asthma and are healthy. Maybe their parents did something that helped. Asthma is seldom outgrown naturally.

Tubercular individuals desire activity, but it is not the only miasm that will exercise. All miasms can be motivated to movement, but for different reasons. Let's consider all of the miasms as they are jogging together. Psora is jogging because she worries about her health and wants to become stronger to protect herself. Sycosis runs to move, compete for first place, win the race and receive attention, and show off. Syphilis runs to escape his depressive thoughts; he'll collapse at the end. Tuberculosis runs because of restlessness and the need for excitement and is in first place for a little while. She is running with her headphones on and the music going, because the exercise is not enough. She will talk and do other things. Patients with the cancer miasm dominant cannot run for long distances.

Many athletes begin life with weakness and work hard to build themselves up to be stronger. At 35 years of age, one may suddenly have a heart attack. I treat some athletes, and in some cases, when I see their x-rays, I see that they are really handicapped people because of all the damage done to their bodies. To me, it is logical that they will die early. They are wearing themselves out. They waste their bodies away with activity day and night.

Slaves in the United States worked very, very hard. Sometimes a ball and chain was placed on the ankles of those slaves who tried to run away. It was torture. It fascinates me to now see people in gymnasiums working out with weights on their legs for exercise! They are running hard, but there is nobody after them, and they are going nowhere! They do this of their own free will. I am reminded of prisoners who in times past were stretched and bent on machines. Working out in gymnasiums today is not the same as the extreme of torture, but we do have nice steel exercise machines with leather or Velcro straps to hold us in. We live in very strange times. Now, with our free will, we are slaves to our passion for fitness. We no longer need to spend our days chopping wood for the fire, hunting for food to feed our families, or turning the soil to grow all of our vegetables and grains. Our lives have become so automated that the need for productive activity and its resultant level of physical fitness has been replaced by working out in gymnasiums, in front of mirrors, worrying about the shapes of our bodies.

Many people who are "slaves" to drugs belong to the tubercular miasm. Always looking for excitement and change, tuberculosis may use cannabis because he wants to escape his normal, boring life. He wants excitement and nice things only to get away from the reality of his life.

In the tubercular miasm and in the tubercular disease, there is a mixture of psoric, sycotic, and syphilitic symptoms because the disease and the miasm are each based on the other three miasms. For example, the weakness and coldness of tuberculosis comes from psora. The need for movement and excitement and the building up of tubercles comes from sycosis. The destruction of the lungs and the spitting of blood are syphilitic. However, the tubercular miasm also has some of its own unique features.

Mental and Emotional Symptoms and Expressions of the Tubercular Miasm

Artistic
Changeable and desiring change
Desire for freedom
Impatience—destructive behavior

Contradictory, changing symptoms
Dictatorial
Delicate, brittle
Excitement—"kicks," then rest, then excitement
Loves travel
Loves the mountains
Needs movement
Oversensitivity to impressions
Creativity—poetry, writing, art, music
Urge to strike or throw
Fear of animals, especially furry ones

A characteristic typical of tubercular people is that they are **oversensitive.** We say that they are oversensitive to all impressions. For this reason, they can produce things that others can't produce, see things that others can't see, and experience things in ways that others can't. Imagine a tubercular painter. He looks at us, goes home, and draws a picture of us. This is his sensitive way of living and feeling. Tubercular people show their feelings in **poetry, writing, and art** and share their feelings openly. They cry, shout, scream. They are sensitive to **music**. Weeping from music belongs to the tubercular (or cancer) miasm.

Another special characteristic of the tubercular miasm is the idea of **travel**. Tubercular people love to travel. Travel includes the **need for movement** found in sycosis with something more added—movement from **place to place**. Tuberculosis feels a need to move his body, his furniture, his home—from one place to another because of an inner drive. He has an irresistible inner drive toward movement that manifests in everything he does: his choice of entertainment, his profession, his relationships. Tuberculosis may **change** his profession every three months, **"traveling" from job to job.** While psora may take a new job to make more money, tuberculosis does this for change and excitement.

Like sycosis, tuberculosis likes **excitement**. It is a very strong symptom of the tubercular miasm. Tubercular people seek out excitement. The "butterflies in the stomach" feeling of excitement is a sycotic/tubercular feeling. Looking for excitement also has the idea of traveling within it. Change is also a kind of travel, and tubercular people want change. They like new studies, new schools, new hobbies. They change jobs, homeopaths, apartments, fashions, partners, and even continents. They are always looking for the **next new thing**. A profession as a pilot or flight attendant would be good for tuberculosis. He can travel throughout his life and smile about it.

Tubercular people enjoy their **freedom**—need their freedom. Without freedom they feel **suffocated.**

When tuberculosis decides to travel, it is quite different from psora's way of travel. Tuberculosis does not need to plan her trip carefully. She simply needs to GO—a spontaneous reaction to the need to move and change. She does not choose to go on a scheduled group trip; that would be too boring. A tubercular person is **impulsive**. She may put all of her things in her rucksack and simply set out, perhaps hitchhiking, working along the way to make a little money. Her way is to do things on impulse. If our close relatives have come from different countries or traveled to many different countries, it brings to mind the possibility of familial tubercular miasm. Of course, we do not understand all the reasons for a person to immigrate to another country, but we do know that the tubercular heritage causes our patients to desire change and movement and excitement.

As long as tuberculosis is involved in a **new thing**, he is energetic. But as soon as he knows his subject well, he quits. A tubercular homeopath will move her practice from one office to another or from one city to another, for a new beginning. When studying her cases, she will move from patient to patient, never able to work on one case for very long. Tuberculosis experiences **many broken relationships** because of "traveling" from one partner to another, needing the excitement of the new. After some time of holding hands with one person, there is not so much excitement anymore. Tubercular people move on. They are never satisfied where they are. They are **easily bored and restless**. They can be self-indulgent and egotistical. They have many **short, intense relationships** and then break off the relationship, rarely achieving deep, strong bonds.

Tuberculosis does aerobics, **runs, jumps, and dances** to loud music. She likes to do a lot of things at the same time. If she can do these things in **open air**, for example, on the top of a mountain, it is perfect for her. Her favorite place is in the **mountains**, where there is fresh air, space, mountains to climb, and a change of scenery from her daily life. Tuberculosis is not happy near the sea. It is too boring for her. Mostly the sea as seen from the shore is flat, with some waves, and that is all.

Tubercular people like **stimulation and excitement**. They do extreme things with their weak bodies. Doing things for **kicks** and excitement can go on throughout the night. They can dance for some time, sometimes without feeling their exhaustion. They don't feel it because they love the movement and the excitement of dancing, but as soon as they are in bed they feel as if they have done too much. All this excitement just does not work well with the condition of their bodies. They may look back with pleasure on what happened, but after the excitement they are **worn out and weak**; they have to rest, then they need more excitement—more rest and then more excitement. This is the life of tubercular people. Sycosis can manage his extremes; he has energy that can last a long time. Tuberculosis does not have as much strength, energy, or endurance as sycosis.

Tuberculosis chooses sports in which she can experience tremendous excitement, for example, bungee jumping. To my mind, it is a stupid thing to jump from a very high place with only a bungee cord separating me from the pavement of the street. The tubercular element craves this kind of excitement. "I can survive it." This is what tuberculosis likes—**exciting sports in open air**. Tuberculosis needs the open air more than her sycotic friends, because she needs the oxygen. Tuberculosis has bursts of energy, but she can **burn out** very quickly. She exhausts herself and at a certain moment gets pneumonia or an illness, and in a few days, she is finished; she has burned herself out.

Tuberculosis is **artistic**. He is often a very good musician. Some tubercular people do not have enough energy to do a lot of exercise, but they have a natural talent for artistic things. These might be children who play the violin at a very young age but never use their capacities to study other things because they are too impatient.

Impatience is another expression of the tubercular miasm. Because she becomes easily and quickly exhausted, her energy is used up and her patience runs out. If something does not go her way, she throws a fit. For example, if she is making a dress and it does not turn out as she wants, she might tear it up, throw it away, or kick it out of the house because she does not have the patience to start again. A psoric person who makes a mistake in knitting or sewing will take it apart and start over.

Tubercular patients also may **destroy** the possessions of others when angry. When she gets upset, she will smash something. She can be aggressive. There is an impulse to **throw or strike**. Sometimes the urge to strike is there even in adults, but adults try to suppress this behavior because it is not socially acceptable. In tubercular children, there is usually throwing and striking, since children are closer to their impulses. Tubercular children have **tantrums**, and tubercular people may engage in unacceptable behavior just for kicks. Some may walk down the street and break things—car antennae, mailboxes—just for fun. This is tuberculosis.

There is **fear of animals** in tuberculosis. Tuberculosis may simply dislike animals; for others, there is true fear. He may say that he is afraid the animals will jump on him and claw him. He is afraid that dogs might bite him. He is especially afraid of cats and other furry animals and does not like the feel of their fur. He may have an allergy to cats. Tuberculosis, as well as sycosis, can kick animals and be cruel to them or even kill them.

Tubercular people are not truly fastidious. They are **impulsive and quick** to react and like excitement and kicks. They are **artistic**, may be **romantic**, and are less likely to be painstaking in their work. They do not have the time to be precise. Their energy is used for the quicker, more exciting parts of living.

General and Physical Symptoms and Modalities of the Tubercular Miasm

Astigmatism
Blue sclera
Bluish skin
Brilliant eyes
Coldness
Contradictory—changing symptoms
Desires cold food and drink, especially milk
Desires fresh air
Emaciates though eats a lot
Elegance in the appearance
Grinds teeth
Inflammation of iris
Low fevers
Needs movement
Narrow—"pigeon" chest (deformity of syphilitic influence)
Physical beauty—"angelic features"—long lashes
Pale shiny skin—high color
Respiratory weakness
Desires rich high-calorie foods—likes fat
Ringworm
Desires smoked foods
Worn out

Many of the characteristic general and physical symptoms of this miasm are similar to the symptoms of the active tubercular disease.

Many of the tubercular patients whom I see are a **little feverish**—with a slightly elevated temperature, never just the average temperature. This is not just when they are sick, but all the time. When they are ill, the body attempts to elevate the temperature, and when they get a high fever, they feel better afterward. They often have night fever. They sweat and perspire from lack of energy, as do psoric patients. They tend to sweat on the chest when they are in bed. They have little stamina and are easily exhausted.

Tuberculosis **emaciates** in her disease. She seems to be wasting away. The tubercular miasm usually produces thin people. The chest is often narrow, with shoulders a bit pronounced, and the sternum and rib cartilage are often prominent. It is called "chicken chest" in Belgium and "pigeon chest" in the United States. This is due to syphilitic deformation of the bones.

Paleness is tubercular. Tubercular people may have a beauty and elegance about them because of the pale delicate skin and sensitive manners. They sometimes get **flushes** (round, red circles) on their cheeks when they get excited, which causes them to look red-faced. A red face in a wasting person is tubercular. The skin may have a blue hue. **Blue sclera** is a tubercular symptom, as is **long eyelashes.**

In the tubercular miasm there is a **weakness in the respiratory system**—breathing problems, allergies, and a tendency to colds. Often there is a history of bronchitis, asthma, and chronic coughs. There is destruction of lung tissue and coughing up of blood. Where there are difficult or recurrent lung problems, the homeopath must always consider the tubercular miasm. Sometimes there will be allergic reactions on the skin and swollen glands.

Tuberculosis cannot cope well with her surroundings. Tubercular people are better in the **mountains** and better in cool or cold air. They love fresh air and cold, dry wind. They are worse heat, rain, or damp.

Tubercular people crave **rich, high-calorie food**. They like pork, bacon, sausage, and fat. They will pick up pieces of fat that psoric *Calcarea carbonica* and *Natrum muriaticum* have left on their plates. Sometimes tuberculosis will eat only the fat and give the meat to somebody else. She really likes this taste, and it gives her needed energy. She likes strong tastes, as does sycosis. Tuberculosis likes all **smoked foods**—fish, meat, and cheese. She is a barbecue specialist, cooking foods outside, "burning" it, smoking it, because she likes that taste. Tuberculosis likes salt. She likes butter and ice cream and likes to drink a lot of cold milk. She **likes cold things**, which is strange for a miasm that generally feels cold. She likes the wind, but not cold air; wind is a kind of excitement, although she will be wrapped up.

When tuberculosis goes to the grocery store, what is at the top of his list? Does he make a list? He wants to buy bacon and ice cream and whatever else excites him at the moment. Tuberculosis may have a big appetite or no appetite. His appetite comes in spurts, but even if he has a big appetite and eats a lot, he can waste away.

The Tubercular Miasm in Infants and Children

When a child is born of parents who have all three miasms or whose ancestors had tuberculosis, the child's behavior will be characteristically tubercular. These "little angels" (and they often look like angels) like fun, and they like new things. They like to touch everything, open everything. When told to stop, they have temper tantrums because they do not like to be told "No." **Temper tantrums** are mostly tubercular. A tubercular child might bang his own head. In the consulting room, they are not as angelic as their physical appearance might suggest.

When I have the chance to treat children adopted from parents in India, Bangladesh, and other parts of Asia, I generally suspect a history of tuberculosis. These children often are given up for adoption because their families are poor, and many of the poor in these countries have this disease. When I see a child who has a history of coughing and who has been treated with antibiotics (mostly a lean, underweight child in the beginning), I am pretty sure this is a tubercular child.

Tuberculosis is **physically beautiful**. This beauty includes **long eyelashes, elegance, refinement** (*Silica* and *Phosphorus* have this), **brilliant eyes, red lips**, and **pale, shiny skin—the angelic look**—all expressions of their delicacy. A deformed, **narrow chest** is the syphilitic influence in the tubercular miasm. In syphilis, deformity takes many forms, in any part of the body. In tubercular patients, the deformity is mostly in the chest, where respiration takes place.

These children are **delicate**, **brittle**, and **irritable**. They need excitement and new things. A psoric child can sit at the table for a long time working puzzles, drawing, and playing, and he is able to finish his activities. Tubercular children jump from one thing to another. One minute they are playing with their cars, then assembling a puzzle, then watching television because the puzzle becomes boring, then painting (they may love to draw and color), then going outside to ride a bicycle. Mostly, they like to be outside. They **change playmates** often. As soon as the excitement is gone, they go to another friend. They are impulsive. They like to play. Many do not want to grow up or be responsible.

They are **dictatorial** with other children and with adults. They can be obstinate and headstrong and not content with their surroundings. A tubercular child can bite and pinch and strike others. There is a bit of violence in them. They can be malicious and spiteful. They also tend to dislike animals.

The tubercular child often sleeps in the **genupectoral** (knees-to-chest) position (*Calcarea phosphorica, Carcinosin, Medorrhinum, Tuberculinum*), as does the sycotic child—on the abdomen, face in the pillow or face pressed on the chest, with knees tucked underneath. She is **restless** and sleepless and sweats, particularly at night on the chest.

Most tubercular children are cold, but a warm child may still need a tubercular remedy.

Children born with the tubercular miasm move a lot, have bronchitis early, and get all manner of coughs and colds. The skin of the tubercular newborn may be **bluish**. The children crave cold milk, but they also may have allergies to milk. Dentition may be slow. They may **grind their teeth** in the night. A tubercular child may have pneumonia—some as early in life as a few months of age, which represents a **child having an adult disease**—a sign of the tubercular or the cancer miasm.

Tubercular Remedies

Tuberculinum is the nosode of the tubercular miasm, but we do not have to use the nosode to treat the miasm. As always, we use the remedies with the strange, rare, and peculiar (SRP) symptoms of the patient that also have a relationship to the prominent miasm of the patient.

There are only two references to "tubercular" in *Kent's Repertory*:

- **HEAD; INFLAMMATION, of; *Brain; tubercular***
- **EYE; INFLAMMATION; *iris; tubercular***

There is no GENERALS "Tuberculosis" rubric in *Kent's Repertory* that provides a reference list of "tubercular" remedies, but we may refer to *Kent's* "Phthisis" rubric for guidance: **CHEST; PHTHISIS *pulmonalis*.**

Modern repertories will have a "Tuberculosis" rubric in the GENERALS section.

For the tubercular miasm, many remedies come to mind:

- *Phosphorus* has a narrow chest, coughing, coughing blood, and the need for excitement.
- *Calcarea phosphorica* loves to travel, is dissatisfied and irritable, and desires smoked meats.
- From professional experience, to *Kent's Repertory* list I would add *Calcarea arsenicosa, Rhus toxicodendron,* and *Kali iodatum* as tubercular remedies.
- *Silica* is not listed in *Kent's Repertory* and yet may be tubercular as well, but it is not as strong a tubercular remedy as some of those listed.

Because we know these remedies well, we can recognize their typical tubercular symptoms. There is very fast movement, a lot of eating yet slimming down, or weakness and exhaustion. All of these are very strong cough remedies. Most remedies have some symptoms of all of the miasms in them. We must look at the prominent symptoms to know how much of the remedy is psoric, sycotic, syphilitic, or tubercular.

A look at the tubercular nosode *Tuberculinum* reiterates these prominent symptoms of the miasm:

- Need for change
- Desire to travel
- Destructiveness, especially when need for change is frustrated
- Fear of animals
- Better in open air
- Better in the mountains
- Marked disposition for respiratory ailments
- Profuse perspiration, at night and from slightest exertion, especially on the chest
- Craving for smoked things, fat, cold milk

Sometimes a case seems blocked: We are sure of the remedy, and yet the indicated remedy does not work. We may have a patient with symptoms of each of the first three miasms plus tubercular symptoms. He may have a lot of fears (psoric), he wakes in the night with the desire to kill his wife (syphilitic), and he has a return of an old gonorrheal discharge (sycotic). He cannot seem to recover his energy, and his glands are swollen (tubercular).

Remember that the tubercular miasm is a combination of psora, syphilis, and sycosis plus its own symptoms. In a case like this, we may be able to give him *Tuberculinum,* and after some time, the case will then clear for further treatment.

Tubercular Case 1: Girl With Allergies, Convulsions, and Tantrums

Video Presentation and Case Description

The following discussion was captured as it occurred during a brief video presentation and case description by Henny Heudens.

This six-year-old child has strong allergic reactions. One grandfather and one aunt have a lot of colds, sinus infections, and heart failure. Two aunts have problems in their ears, and the mother is allergic in the same way as the little girl. On the father's side, the grandfather has a lot of bronchitis, and an uncle has many colds. During the pregnancy, the child was not expected with joy. The parents' relationship was difficult. The mother was ready to break it off when she was told she was pregnant. They split up when the baby was one-and-a-half years old. The mother was ill from the first three months until the end of the pregnancy with a lot of diarrhea and swollen glands on the right side of her neck. The baby was breastfed for six months and received support formula for another two months. A lot of vomiting occurred during the six months of breastfeeding.

At one year of age, the child had convulsions during a fever, and when she was one-and-a-half years old, the parents separated. When she had fever and convulsions, she was given antibiotics. The convulsions were quite strong, and the mother is afraid she will get other fevers now since she is not that healthy.

When I see the child for the first time the mother is in a new relationship. The child does not accept the boyfriend. We see this very often when a mother has been alone with a child for some time. The child gets jealous and becomes aggressive. This little girl has acted aggressively not only since she met her mother's boyfriend but also before this. About nine months ago (about four to five months before the new boyfriend came into the picture), she started throwing herself on the floor, beating her fists, kicking, and breaking and throwing things. About 14 months before this consultation, the mother lived with another boyfriend. She had to work a lot to provide money for the child, and various people cared for the child—a neighbor, an aunt, the grandmother. When the mother lived with her second boyfriend, again there were several caretakers for the little girl while the mother was at work.

How is the child's situation? First the parents split up, and then the mother starts to live with her boyfriend. That relationship ends, and now the mother starts a new relationship. During this time, the child becomes more and more aggressive. The child does not allow the new boyfriend to be in the consulting room.

Let's watch this child for a while. What is your feeling/response to the child? Do you like the child? I find her very feminine. The mother is a very nice lady—polite and well educated. What is the child doing? [*Coloring left-handed.*] I gave her pencils and crayons to draw and noticed she was left-handed. We do not have remedies that are left-handed or right-handed, but being left-handed is less common—perhaps we could think of it as reversed?

Another patient of mine had a chest that was "reversed." His heart was on the right side, and his organs were totally reversed. He was healthy except for allergies. Having his heart on the right side is syphilitic because it is a kind of deformation. If a child develops left-handedness, there is something in his heritage that makes him do something in a way that is opposite or uncommon. He is creating an action using the side of the brain opposite the norm. It is a syphilitic sign. Have you ever thought about it? It means that in the family where this happens, someone in the past had syphilis and suppressed it. It is a hint from the vital force. When one develops teeth, the front teeth usually come in first. Is it wrong for the canines to emerge first? No, not at all. It is a minor characteristic, but for homeopaths it is a sign that there is something in the child's development that is not orderly. People who are left-handed also have a little bit of that. It is a hint for the miasm, and we must notice all signs given by the vital force that some process is at work. Merely being left-handed does not mean that someone's great-great grandfather had syphilis, but it is possible.

Signs and symptoms of abnormal development are a hint that the syphilitic miasm is present in the case to some degree.

So—teeth that emerge out of order, or left-handedness, or kidneys in an unusual place in the body, or heart on the right side instead of the left, or people who have one brown eye and one blue, all have a kind of exotic quality, but all are from the same inherited miasm (syphilis).

The mother is talking about the child's fever; it gets high quickly. The child talks softly, shyly to the mother, not to me. This child traveled a great distance by train to come to the consultation. I like her. She is not interested in me at all or at least does not act interested. She watches herself on the screen.

The mother tells that the child has been very headstrong and stubborn since she was three years old. She has always been distant, not a child who cuddled mom or liked to be kissed a lot. Observe her after 14 hours of travel and compare her to the boy we saw yesterday. She is curious, not mischievous like he was. Now she is drawing again. The first complaint is aggression. The second complaint is convulsions, with redness and heat. During the convulsions, she makes movements with her arms as if striking or beating someone. Her eyes turn upward. The mother is very afraid of the convulsions, but she trusts the boyfriend, who believes in homeopathy.

The third complaint is allergies to a lot of foods: carrots, apples, pears, hazelnuts (definitely), and others. She reacts with swelling, tears, and eye pain. She has been experiencing these allergic reactions for one-and-a-half years. This painful reaction lasts from two to three hours, and then the pain subsides, although the swelling remains for a few days.

The mother is also shy, very nice, thin, delicate, refined. I know she is a very sensitive lady, with a lot of problems because of the child's behavior. She cannot imagine why the child behaves this way. She tries to correct her in a loving way, but the child does not respond and throws tantrums.

The child bites her nails, has a lot of colds, and gets throat infections. She gets pain in the throat and coughing, and then the fever starts. She likes to play with dolls. She has the restlessness and motion of the boy we saw yesterday. She is looking around, playing with the pencils, and changing position a lot. She liked traveling by train because she could walk around in it, and the mother had a lot of toys for her. For some minutes, she would play with the games, and then after a while, she only wanted to play with the mother. The mother is a loving mother and looks sad. The child tells her she wants to leave the consultation because she is bored.

The daycare workers say she behaves fine. At home, there is a difference. She loves sweets and pancakes, and heat gives her a headache in the front of her head. She is not cold. She drinks very little, sleeps well, talks in her sleep, grinds her teeth, picks her nose and eats it, and has a lot of accidents because her mind gets confused and she forgets to watch what she is doing. She bruises herself because of imprudence. She loves milk products. In bed, she has fear of robbers. That is the whole case.

The mother says that although the child is on her lap, this is not usual. The girl is hiding herself from me. She does not want to be observed.

Tubercular Case 1—Analysis

How do we analyze this case to get the remedy? We have some syphilis in the case. [*She has a duality in her personality. We see her shyness, but there is also the aggressiveness at home.*] When parents tell us these things, can we trust it? Of course, parents do not like to tell bad things about their children because they love them. If parents come to homeopathy, they are desperate and frustrated with allopathy. Why do some parents come to homeopathy and some do not? Some think more deeply about their children's health. They look more into the future and are willing to use long-term treatment.

What else is there in addition to the split in the personality? [*Tantrums, aggressiveness, throwing herself, violence.*] In such a sweet nice, well-educated child, we see violence that is spontaneous, but not evil or premeditated.

What do you feel for this child? As you gain experience with patients you become more sensitive to what is not spoken and to what you are feeling in yourself during the interview. To differentiate your own "symptoms" from those of the patient you must know yourself very well. If you know you are characteristically quickly irritated and you get irritated because a child touches your book, it is *your* symptom. If you are *not* quickly irritated and you get irritated when a child touches your book, it is a symptom from the *child.* The child brings it out in you. For example, I am quite optimistic by nature. Depressive feelings are uncharacteristic of me except when I go to the waiting room, call my next patient, and the patient is very depressed. Between the waiting room and my consulting room, I feel emotionally heavier. I feel some of their depression and take it in. This change in my own emotion is a sign for me of how deep a patient's depression is even without hearing one word. Yesterday, when the child simply touched my book, I felt irritated with him because of how he did it. Use these things to know your patients.

Have you ever felt danger in your consulting room when you are not normally very afraid? Once, even though I am usually not suspicious at all, I left my consulting room to get a remedy for a patient while she remained in the room. I went down the stairs, but went back up right away because I sensed something out of the ordinary for me and found her stealing my money. She had the money in her hand. I asked, "What are you doing?" She said, "I lost something." When you feel something about your patients that causes you fear or gives you a sense of danger, look for dangerous remedies.

I like this girl, even though her mother tells of her bad behavior. What is another of her symptoms? [*Sudden high fever with convulsions.*] What is unusual about her convulsions? [*That she strikes during the convulsions.*] What does she express to me? There is a kind of playfulness; she does not want to like me, but it is not really that bad. If she were older, you would call it flirtatious. She moves a lot, even though she is very tired from her travel. She is gentle, gracious, and very feminine. See how she is playing with the shawl. She is hiding herself, then exposing herself, moving a lot, showing a lot of restlessness. She looks as if she'd like to settle down, but she can't. She is entertaining herself. She is very artistic. Is she enjoying anything in the movement? Yes, she is enjoying herself. She lives her own life. I like the idea that if she were older, she would be flirting. There is a certain self-confidence; she is self-contained. She does not seem to care about her mother or me. I feel that she thinks she is pretty.

I did not think of sexual abuse in this child. When children have a history of sexual abuse, sometimes there is a kind of closing up, not liking to expose themselves because that can be dangerous; or one may observe the contrary, a lot of exposure in an almost sexual way. In those two extremes, I might be thinking that something sexual happened to the child. This child is still innocent, although there is some precocity. I have the feeling she can tease or toy with people. This is somewhat advanced for a six-year-old.

What is another characteristic of the child? [*Allergies.*] There is discharge from the eyes, swelling, pain and inflammation and burning, and she grinds her teeth at night. She has accidents, but not from lack of coordination. Her coordination is fine. She is impulsive, is too quick, and does not see the danger. [*How about the mother's lack of joy at being pregnant?*] How was the mother? Swollen glands and tired until the end of the pregnancy. She is a nice, delicate mother. From what family background is the child coming? Tubercular.

Now we come to the remedy she needs. We have a gracious child, precocious, grinding teeth, desires milk, tantrums, tubercular illnesses in the family and in pregnancy, the mother having tubercular characteristics herself—moving a lot, curious, restless. This is a *Tuberculinum* child who comes from a mother with a tubercular background and a tubercular shape. The mother has the syphilitic shape in her face. The face and chin are elongated and thin, and the chin protrudes. There is something wrong in the way the two jaws work together. There are also allergic reactions in the child's background—a grandfather with bronchitis, colds, and sinusitis. This is the place where the tubercular miasm likes to cause problems.

Now do we understand why the child is left-handed? The tubercular miasm is made up of psora, syphilis, and sycosis. Because there is syphilis in the pot, a tubercular patient will also exhibit syphilitic symptoms or expressions. They are gracious and charming but not connected as syphilis is disconnected. This is why they move a lot, change jobs a lot, travel around, and are never able to settle down. We see this movement in the little child, even as tired as she is. What is the difference between the disconnection of *Mercury* and *Tuberculinum*? She is connected to herself and can feel quite happy with herself. She is not content with her surroundings. She needs new things, new toys, new fashions. She always needs more kicks. When she is older, she will be playful with people instead of with her pencils and crayons. She will become bored with new relationships, not because she is bad, but because she is tubercular. Her mother has this behavior. Without the remedy, the child might run away from home and not be able to settle down. With boys, she could have one relationship after another, perhaps two or three at a time. After her remedy, the first result will be to get more strength and more connection to the mother, be more contented, and be able to concentrate. She will be able to deal with this natural feeling of beauty. She may be an artist.

What kind of artist might she be after homeopathy? She may dance or draw or maybe do homeopathy. She will be more able to find satisfaction in her work; she will not always be looking for something else to satisfy her. Her future will be much better.

[*When the boy we saw yesterday cut up the picture, I thought this was a tubercular thing.*] This girl can do the same thing, but for her it is more impulsive. The boy wanted to worry the mother, to threaten, so to speak, that he was going to do it. *Tuberculinum* does this kind of thing because they have a great need for kicks, stimulation, and excitement. When we get angry, what happens? [*Adrenaline.*] What do we do with this? If we are quite healthy, although we may feel we would like to kick and hit, we do not, because we can control it. When tubercular people are angry, they cannot control it. They do not have the power. They can get into trouble in life this way.

Tuberculinum has fear of robbers also, even though it is not listed in the Repertory for that rubric. [*Fear like in Natrum muriaticum?*] Yes. She gets headaches from the heat, and *Tuberculinum* loves cold air and wind. The wind represents excitement and change for the tubercular person. What other N*atrum muriaticum* symptoms do we have? [*Refined, self-contained, looks nice.*] Yes, but if I showed you *Natrum muriaticum* children, you would see a very different atmosphere. Let's see her followup now.

Tubercular Case 1—Followups

At this three-month followup, she is hiding less. She has been coughing very badly for one month. She needs some water to get over the cough. Immediately after the remedy, she was fine. Very quickly, she started to speak with her mother's boyfriend and make contact with him. Her headache was soon better. She developed a high fever for one day without convulsions, and after the fever she had much less aggressive behavior. After the first visit to see her father she became aggressive again, and then she started this cough a month ago as if she had whooping cough, a barking cough. With all children who have to alternate between visiting two parents, my homeopathic mind says this is very difficult for them, even though I know they need to have both parents in their lives.

She has had a fever now for three days of about 101 degrees F and a dramatic cough. We see her because she is ill and is in an acute situation. We have to find out whether she has had a relapse. There was a return of some symptoms after a visit to the father: She became aggressive, with coughing and fever but without convulsions. She is more aggressive toward the boyfriend again. [*Is this because of the fever or the visit to the father?*] That is what I am asking you. What must we do?

Children are always loyal to their parents. I love this about children. It is uncommon for children to talk about things that their parents do to hurt them. If they do reveal such things, we must take it seriously because it is unusual for children to talk about such matters. I hear a lot of fear from children who know other children who have gone through a divorce; they do not want this for themselves. I know of many children who give other children advice about their parents' splitting up. Many illnesses come with the etiology of divorce.

What do we do? We take the case again. Do not get stuck with the cough and fever. She plays normally, dancing with the doll to show the camera. She sleeps without fear. She was eating and drinking normally, until now. She has had swollen eyes after eating apples but can eat carrots without any reaction. She is irritable in the morning when she gets up; she is easily irritated and not as angry anymore with her mother but sometimes angry with the boyfriend. She beats him and pinches him. The preschool gives very good reports about her. This is her case. [*Drinking something ameliorates the cough?*] Yes, we see this. She is coughing in spells—a choking cough. [*Is this rage normal, or is it due to a relapse?*] This is our question, and we always have to be sure of the answer when managing our cases.

A typical situation is that we see the patient back after his remedy, and we have to know whether the remedy worked initially and whether it is still working or whether a symptom or set of symptoms points to a relapse. In the consulting room, we usually have to figure this out alone. Now we can discuss this together. [*I can see myself giving a low potency of the same remedy. Things are moving in the right direction.*]

Let's take the possibilities:

- We can repeat.
- We can go higher or lower.
- We can wait a while longer and give nothing.
- We can give a new remedy.

Which of you would like to repeat? [About one-third.] Who likes to go higher? [Nobody.] Who likes to go lower? [Three people.] Who likes to do nothing? [Many people.] Who likes to give a new remedy? [Nobody.] So we have two possibilities. Was the remedy working? [*Yes.*] What did the remedy do? [*Aggression decreased very much.*] What else? [*Emotional improvement.*] [*No more convulsions even with high fever; restlessness better.*] [*Better connection with boyfriend and then relapse.*] [*Eating and drinking are better.*]

I had the feeling when I saw her back for this followup that her face looked more pronounced, with her hair pulled back. Look at the video. She looks as if she has gained weight. She looks more like a child and less like a woman. The precocious behavior isn't there anymore. She looks more childlike, more her own age in the way she plays and behaves. She was clearly better until this moment, except for the fever for three days and the cough for one month. How is the cough disturbing her? [*Not much. She does not seem to be asking for help that much. The cough wouldn't bother me so much except for the emotional symptoms coming back. I have a problem with that.*] What kind of symptom is the cough? [*Tubercular.*] What else are cough and fever in the history? [*A recurrent thing.*] Yes, before with the fever, she had convulsions. If she is getting back an old symptom, even when it is coughing, it is good. Everything else is better. She looks well. [*Her energy is still okay, but she is aggressive again with the boyfriend.*] Yes, this is still a difficulty.

I suggest making a small list to better visualize the situation. For example, certain things are much better, and certain symptoms have returned. If I repeat her remedy, I am not sure I am doing the correct thing. I only like to do something when I am sure. When you repeat a remedy too early, what could be the result? You could lose in one or two days much or all you have accomplished.

The principle is to WAIT if you are not sure. If you do not give a remedy, things will get either better or worse; things will not remain the same.

Is the child in danger? Not at all. When you feel you do not know what to do, the best thing to do is to wait. Let your patient contact you by phoning back in one day or one week to see how the case develops. When you see that she is worse and that she stops eating or sleeping, it means her energy level has gone down. That would be a clear indication to repeat the remedy. I asked the mother to wait and to call me if the child becomes worse. I did not get a phone call.

[*Would you ever give Tylenol for the fever?*] In some cases perhaps, but not in this case. She had a lower fever and did not even get a convulsion with the high fever. Be logical about this.

[*She's angry with the boyfriend and not with everyone else anymore.*] Yes, this is more appropriate. Everything is so much better. We know she is stronger; she is not as delicate anymore. She is in a better situation to stand fever. My only doubt is whether she is strong enough to overcome the cough now.

[*What if she gets a convulsion now? Would this be a sign that this is the wrong remedy?*] She is better on all levels, even with the allergic reactions. We know it is the right remedy. I am convinced that when she has a relapse that tells us what she needs, we will repeat the remedy. We have proof that it worked beautifully.

We had another followup six months after the initial consult. Look at the video and watch how she is. She is playing, focused on the game in her lap. She is disconnected from me again. Her expression is not happy. She coughed for two more weeks after the last appointment, but the day after I saw her it became less severe. When the cough was gone, she got a throat infection with a high fever for two days but no side effects. In February, after a visit to her father's house, she behaved very badly. She could not sleep, was very restless, and was kicking and hitting her mother. They phoned me. High fever—bad behavior—restlessness. I repeated the remedy at that point.

When a repeat dose is needed, give the same potency that gave the good response. Only go higher when the same potency does not work anymore.

Then she started to cough and had a low fever. This is exactly the same reaction as before. Her behavior improved. After the third day of fever, she was very aggressive toward the boyfriend. She told him while kicking him, "Now I will kill you." He said to her, "Why?" She said, "I don't want a whole series of fathers." He said, "Why do you think you'll get a whole series of fathers?" "First one, then another one, now you, then another one; I will kill every father that comes in my house." She is expressing her problem now. He took her on his lap, and she fought him. He said, "Listen, you may fight and leave my lap, but I want you to be here only one minute, and then you can do what you like." He told her that he loved her mother and that he loved her and said, "I promise I will never leave you." She cried, went to her room for a long time, and then went to her mother. She asked her mother whether her mother loved him and whether she would leave *him.* The mother was shocked because she wasn't as sure as the boyfriend was. She realized what the child was going through. She told the child that if she ever thought of leaving him, she would talk to the child first. The child then went back to him and said, "Can you play with me?" The relationship has been fine since then. She dealt with the problem. She was coughing and choking before, possibly because she could not express how she felt.

Now I see this little girl who turns her back on me and does not want to talk to me. What have I to do? I take the case and hear that she is much happier: has almost no allergic reactions, no longer bites her nails, has no reaction to nuts, likes to play outside, sometimes has difficulty playing alone, took a toy out of a shop once without paying but went back to apologize. She sleeps very well and talks in her sleep. She still eats stuff out of her nose but has fewer accidents and is better after the weekends with her father. This is a good report, but I see a child who turns away from me, who does not like the consultation.

How are children with consultations? Some love them—to talk about themselves, to hear bits and pieces of conversation about them, to play with the toys—but many children do not like them at all. This child had to hear her mother tell, in front of the camera, about her stealing something. When children six years old do not like talking about or hearing about their mistakes or faults, do they need a remedy? No. She has to come to understand that stealing is unacceptable behavior and that one must fix the mistake if possible, but none of us likes to hear our mistakes talked about in the consulting room. I did not do anything after this consultation. When a child does not like the consultation, does that constitute a relapse? She now is playing nicely by herself. The mother says she is more affectionate now. Two doses of *Tuberculinum* so far. She is putting the little cars in a certain order, from small to big. She puts things in order. She left the toys in good order when she and her mother departed.

The next followup is two months later: Now she can eat carrots (though not too many), salad, everything, without any reaction. She is a much calmer child. The coughing has stopped. New symptoms include skin peeling on the tips of the fingers and a fungus on her toe. There is no aggression at all. Her mother tells me that the child is the "police-child" of the family. She is bossy, telling how everything should be done, and the mother is not very happy about that because the child does not instruct people in a polite way. She is fine with her mother's boyfriend. Her appetite is fine, and she has no headaches, although she can be angry when she does not get something she wants. There is no grinding of teeth or eating stuff out of her nose, and her sleep is fine.

I ask the mother, "What do you want the homeopathic remedy to do now?" She tells, "Make her not so bossy." The little girl is very proud about the flower in her hair when I tell her I like it. We wait. All of her symptoms are gone except those on the skin, and she is growing up. She is trying to cope with getting bigger. We do not do anything about the fungus for the foot. She will get a remedy for the fungus only when there is a relapse or when a totally new picture emerges for a totally new remedy. Do not use allopathic thinking in doing something for the fungus.

Why did she get a fungus? [*Her susceptibility.*] People are always trying to treat fungus. When fungus is on the nails and the patient is fine, why is it there? It is an eruption on the skin, a discharge; this means there is still a bit of weakness. When she is strong, her body will avoid the fungus.

What if people come to you for the treatment of fungus? Take the case and see what is needed.

Tubercular Case 2: Man With Prostatitis

Video Presentation and Case Description

The following discussion was captured as it occurred during a video presentation and case description by Henny Heudens. Henny's comments during the video are in parenthesis. Student questions and comments appear within brackets. In the interview portions, "HH" indicates a question or comment by Henny, and "P" indicates comments or responses of the patient.

I saw this patient in front of a class of homeopaths. His homeopathic doctor was with him. The patient has a diagnosis of essential prostatitis. He has been given 50 homeopathic remedies, including *Sulphur*, *Kali bichromicum*,

Berberis, China, Medorrhinum, Thuja, Lycopodium, Kali carbonicum, Pulsatilla, Causticum, Mercury, Syphilinum, Psorinum, Calcarea, and many smaller remedies. His father had stomach problems, gout, and some strange palpitations of the heart (disturbances in the rhythm). His mother had no problems. One paternal uncle had epilepsy, and another uncle with lung disease died at age 22 years. His grandfather died very young (at 40 years of age) of an unknown disease. The maternal grandmother died at 84 years of age. His father also died at 84. One paternal uncle had heart disease and died at 70 years of age. The paternal grandmother had vein disease and heart disease. There is no cancer in the family, but there are heart and lung diseases.

This man is younger than 40 years old and is the only child in the family. His homeopath gave a complete history. He has a burning feeling in his testicle, sometimes a gripping feeling and sometimes a pinching feeling. He suffers from pain in his kidneys or in the kidney region of the back. He has a constant urge to urinate. We might think of *Sepia* (always the feeling of "having to go"), especially if this were a female patient. He said he had diarrhea and then began experiencing pressure in the bladder. He first had complaints in his intestines that finished after a few days, followed by the feeling of always having to urinate (he has had this for two-and-a-half years.). Now there is gripping pain in the testicle that burns and presses. In the hospital, they examined his kidneys and x-rayed the kidneys and bladder, finding no obstruction. They examined his prostate gland and did an ultrasound. He had gotten sick in August and had antibiotics for two months with no results. They took sperm, and everything was negative, although there was some staphylococcus.

The man is telling about all his misery and how he was given antibiotics many times. His pain and problems are still there. How is he? [*Loquacious. He gives a very detailed account of his symptoms.*] He gives a full explanation of all the details. [*He looks quite healthy.*] He is young, is not married, has no children, and looks healthy. [*He looks like he's in control of everything.*] His profession is managing a big store where 20 people sell clothing. He wears a very nice sweater. In his job, he dresses in a suit. [*He looks closed.*] Yes, he wants to control. He is anxious about me. He has sharp eyes, small glasses. His sickness started in August, so my question was, what happened in August? He was on holiday, and he likes to swim. The water was very cold, and after the first swim, he got a pain in the abdomen and diarrhea. The diarrhea finished in two days, and then the pressure started on his bladder.

HH— Was this the first time you suffered this?

P—Well, I had this problem for the first time in August, but I think I am quite sensitive to swimming in cold water. Once when I was young, I had to do some exercise in cold water and developed a cough afterward. (His pullover is warm for my consulting room, and he shows no sign of it being too warm.)

HH—How were your holidays? Did something else happen? Why did you choose this place for your holiday?

P—I go every year because I like to be alone in the mountains. I see so many people in the shop where I work, so I like quiet holidays; it helps me cope with people. (I want to find out whether he always likes to be alone.)

HH—Do you live alone?

P—Yes.

HH—Since when?

P—For some years.

HH—Why do you live alone?

P—Because you can't always live with your parents.

HH—Have you ever thought of having a family?

P—No. All my friends are married, and I see such a lot of trouble in their relationships. When you build up your life, buy your apartment, buy nice things, get married, and the woman leaves in three years, I don't want to do that. I prefer to be free.

HH—So you prefer not to be in a relationship?

P—Not fanatically. I have a girlfriend.

HH—Why wasn't she with you on holiday?

P—I had met her only three weeks before the holiday. She had already arranged hers, and I had arranged mine; next year, perhaps she will go with me. (He tells us very little so far. He is really very closed.)

HH—By this age you have probably had some relationships? How many?

P—Let me count. What do you mean by a relationship?

HH—Most people mean a sexual relationship. How many have you had?

P—Uh, two.

HH—What happened with those relationships?

P—Well, you know. You are a woman. You know what the world is like. As soon as they go out with you and they hear you have an apartment and a nice car and are the only child of the family, they immediately want to marry. I told you already I don't want to marry.

It is important to know about a patient's sexual relationships when he has prostate problems. It could be a sexual disease, but with him, it does not seem so at this point. Look at the video. He looks as if he is expecting me to punish him with my questions. He sits in a protective position. I feel as if he is expecting me to hurt him. What can we use so far? [*He is suspicious. People could take away his apartment, his car.*] Yes, how much does he really have? At this age, European people do not usually have their own apartment. He probably has money from his parents.

HH—How is your relationship with your parents?

P—Good, very good.

HH—How often do you see your parents? He tells me that he spends Monday evenings with his parents; on Saturdays he works until 6:00 P.M. and then goes to his parents' house for dinner. Then he goes out with friends or his girlfriend. Sunday he sleeps late, and then he has dinner and sleeps at his parents' house. He goes to a movie in the evening. He says, "When I am working, I sleep in my apartment." For me, this implies that he is with his parents too much for his age. There is strong dependency.

HH—Do you cook for yourself?

P—Oh no, my mother cooks for me, and I heat it in the oven. If not, I go to a restaurant; I don't prepare meals myself.

HH—What do you like to eat? (He looks to heaven to get the answers.)

P—I like caviar and oysters, and I can't miss a glass of wine with my dinner.

HH—Do you drink wine every day?

P—Yes, after a long day of work I eat a good, well-prepared meal and drink one to three glasses of wine. Before going to sleep, I drink the rest of the bottle of wine.

This is unusual in Belgium. Belgians might have some wine with dinner on Sunday; oysters and caviar are not things we eat weekly, only for celebrations. He looks to heaven for the answers again. He is very uncomfortable with the question and tries to gain time. If he still smoked, he would light up a cigarette slowly to gain time to think about his answers. He likes to give his answers precisely, to give the correct answer without doubt. He tries to make a good impression. This is a psoric feeling. He wants people to think good things about him.

He has fear of losing his possessions, and he is very cold. These are psoric things. What does he like in foods? [*Rich foods.*] This belongs to the psoric miasm. I cannot understand why such a healthy-looking person who jumps into the water would get this colic. Most people jump in and get right out. Something is weak, but he does not look weak.

HH—Did something else happen before the holiday?

P— No, afterward. Well, it was not a nice homecoming for me.

HH—Why not?

P—I got home in the evening and had to work the next day. I knew that the big boss of all the international shops had retired during my holiday and that in the next week a new director would be named. I am the best, so everybody expected me to be this country's chief. The evening I returned from vacation, I went to the letterbox to see all my mail, and there was a letter from the company telling me that Mr. So-and-So had been named director.

HH—How did you react?

P—I got angry because I didn't get that job, and I picked up the phone and privately called another person who had helped choose the new director. I shouted at him, "I have worked for you for 13 years from 7:00 in the morning (instead of the usual arrival time of 8:30 A.M.) and went home at 7:00 P.M. when I could have gone home at 6:00 P.M. At noon, I only had a sandwich so I could supervise, and now you do this to me!" Then I couldn't sleep all night, and that night for the first time I felt the pain in the testicle.

Is there any connection here? [*Yes.*] What did he go through? [*Disappointment.*] Who has not gone through disappointment? The disappointment is not the symptom, but his pain in the testes after anger is unusual. How was his anger? [*Rage.*]

Can you imagine being the employee and phoning the responsible person to shout at him because you were not chosen? Violent anger toward a superior is unusual in Belgium. So this is a symptom. We need to find a remedy that has all these kinds of things. After the pain in the testicle, the illness went on as described.

HH—What did you do the next day?

P—I had to work. I decided that, queue or no queue (traffic), I would leave in just enough time for work so that I would be a bit late. The other workers wouldn't be able to get in, and I wanted the people to see that the company had really hurt me by not giving me the position of chief. I was three-quarters of an hour late, and everybody was anxious that I might have had an accident because this had never happened before. I explained to the girls how the company behaved toward me and how the boss had behaved. I told them I would come for my job on time and leave at the exact time at night. (Some had thought that perhaps he was shy. Is this shy? [*No*].)

HH—Were you afraid you would lose your job?

P—No, I have arranged insurance so that I can't lose my job.

HH—What kind of insurance is this?

P—You know, I was not really sure about the job, so before I left on holiday I joined the union. I never did this before because it cost money, but the law is that when you work for a long time in a job and are a member of the union and are terminated, they have to pay you three years' salary. This is my insurance. I get my money, I am free, and they have to pay. (This is very clever, insuring his future beforehand. He was making his money safe for the future.)

Tubercular Case 2—Analysis

To what miasm does this case belong? [*Psora.*] Patients do not ordinarily say that they have fear of the future. They tell their history, and we must discern what is strange, rare, and peculiar. We have found his miasm. This is a psoric patient. He has to be sure about the future, works hard in a job that he has had for a long time, sees his boss as an enemy, takes the union as the big brother to help him, and desires rich food. What is behind the psora? [*Heart and lung problems.*] We need a remedy for:

- A cold person
- A fastidious person
- An angry person
- Pains pressing down
- Desire for wine and expensive, rich food
- Idea of marriage unendurable
- Pain in prostate

I gave him *Nux vomica* 200C. When my class discussed this case, some of them eliminated *Nux vomica* because he had no stomach problems. This is clinical thinking.

Nux vomica is listed in plain type under all the miasms. He gets *Nux vomica* 200C because he is strong. He has a good vital force. I could have given higher, but what do I really know about this case? It is not strong miasmatically, but he is somewhat strong. When I know patients will need more remedies, I do not like to give potencies that are too high. Many patients who are treated by homeopaths with remedies in high potencies become weak and tired, not strong. I am very careful not to overprescribe. The way he behaves with his boss is not typically psoric, but we do know it belongs to *Nux vomica.* It is a sycotic reaction, a strong heavy reaction. *Nux vomica* is also listed under **GENERALS; SYCOSIS**.

It is probably better to give a lot of remedies that are totally wrong than a remedy or series of remedies that are close to the simillimum, because the patient will not react to remedies if they are not close enough—not similar to his state. The sensitive patient reacts to everything, and some patients are so sensitive that they react to almost any remedy taken. When a patient does not react to an incorrect remedy, this mostly shows a strong vital force.

Tubercular Case 2—Followups 1 and 2

He came back for a followup in three months. His homeopath did not want me to wait too long to treat. She was afraid he might have cancer. She phoned me to say that the remedy did not do anything. (We had an agreement to see him back in six months in front of the group). In the second consultation (first followup), his kidney pain was much better, and his back was better. His problems at work were gone, and he felt fine. He had decided that he would do his job. He had testicular pain sometimes and sometimes not, and the bladder was the same. Is the remedy working? [*Yes. Back pain is better, social problems are better, testicular pain is changing.*] He tells me that he has gotten used to the pain. We decided to wait and see what would happen in the next few months.

After three more months (second followup), he does not look so closed anymore; he is more himself. He looks relaxed after holiday. Sometimes he is better and sometimes worse. At certain moments, he has pain. The pain has been totally gone for 10 to 14 days, and now it is back. He says:

P—After I last saw you, I got an aggravation here in my back. Now I feel worried about something. I once had a spontaneous pneumothorax and was in the hospital, and I feel this same pain now in my upper back. You know, during my holidays I started to cough because of swimming in the cold water.

He went to his allopathic doctor when he returned from his holiday and was given antibiotics for his cough. In the past two weeks, the pain came back, with pressure on the bladder.

What did the doctor try to suppress? [*His symptoms, his cough.*] This stopped the row of falling dominoes. The symptoms relapsed. Now the pain was paralyzing; he could not bend down or turn in the chair.

P—I could only lie down. This is exactly how I felt years ago. I was anxious about it because it took me weeks to get over it before. The cough had stopped, but now it is coming back. I feel weak, and the cough is coming back.

I asked whether he had pain with sex, and he said no. He has dry spots on his skin, drinks a little coffee, coke, and tea. He cut down the amount of wine to two glasses. He now starts to eat ice cream, and his temperature has gone up slightly. He is a little feverish and perspires during the night. There is a return of old symptoms, and we are happy when that happens.

What is he doing in his reaction? How is his vital force expressing what he needs? He has fear, goes to the doctor, and takes antibiotics, and now the pain is greater, and the fever remains. What did the antibiotics do? [*Blocked his energy.*]

His homeopathic doctor had already given him another dose of *Nux vomica,* and there was no reaction. What do we have to do? Does he need another remedy? Normally, when you are in good shape and your energy is coping and an old symptom comes back, you feel better in spite of the old symptom. His old symptom came back, but he feels weak and feverish. Is there improvement anymore, and does he need the same remedy?

Points to consider:

- His general temperature went up, and he is craving ice cream and sweating at night.
- *Nux vomica* usually does not crave ice cream.
- He is feverish, needing open air. Here we come to the interesting point. He had two problems in the family in the past: heart and lung problems. He has the tubercular miasm in his past.
- When we first saw him, he was psoric. And now?
- *[Tubercular.]* Yes, now he needs a tubercular remedy. He needs *Tuberculinum.*

HH—When you were ill and you needed to see the doctor, what did you do?
P—I called for the doctor to visit me because I was too weak to go to him.
HH—Where were you when you were ill and called for the doctor?
P—In my apartment.
HH—Did someone care for you or help you?
P—No. I didn't need any food, and I didn't want my mother with me because she is always so anxious and always caresses me so much. I could never bear this when I was so ill.

Reasons for *Tuberculinum:*

- Needs a tubercular remedy
- Desires ice cream
- Desires fresh air
- Did not want his mother (against psora)

He did not get pneumonia—he got an old symptom less severe than before. The vital force needed to clear the background of his family disease. He needed to cough again and get fever to be able to tell the homeopath he did not need *Nux vomica* anymore. Why not? How is *Nux vomica* with fresh air when he is feverish? *Nux vomica* cannot even have his blanket off a little because he is so cold. This patient craves fresh air and desires ice cream. This is against *Nux vomica.* He has his old pain back. I was sure of what he needed because the vital force spoke his language, and I observed it.

Tubercular Case 2—Third Followup

He came back one month later because his homeopath wanted him to come. He looks psoric again. He is back to his beginning state, perhaps like the first consultation. He looks to the ceiling; he puts his finger in his mouth. He looks more timid and a little bit sad. I get a report from his homeopath that he got rid of the cough very soon after the *Tuberculinum.* His fever was gone, and he went on a planned holiday with his girlfriend to be at the marriage of his friend. He and his girlfriend were the witnesses, which means they are getting closer. They are accepted as a couple. He is not quite as fearful of marriage. They found the wedding they attended to be so beautiful that they are now planning their own marriage. He got heart palpitations going home on the plane, which made him nervous because his grandfather died from heart disease. He showed me the prescription for Valium and other drugs. They discovered his blood pressure was high. His homeopath was afraid the *Tuberculinum* had caused heart disease, but what kind of palpitation was this? He had tests in the hospital, and they said he was only a little nervous. They told him, "Quiet yourself a little, take some Valium, sleep well, and your blood pressure and palpitations will go away. If it does not go away, you can take these prescriptions to calm you down." If you treat with homeopathy correctly, the reaction will be less severe than with allopathic drugs. He is just a little anxious, but instead of feeling it in the testicle and in the lungs or back, he feels it in his heart.

Many people who fall in love feel palpitations in their hearts. When disappointed in love, people say that they feel like their hearts are broken, which is a syphilitic reaction. What is his reaction? Psoric. What would be the reaction with sycosis? Tachycardia or an enlarged heart.

The problem was not structural with him, just nerves, which goes along with the nervousness and timidity. What did he need? A dose of *Nux vomica,* and this was the end of his case. In 13 months, the chronic prostatitis was cured. Is this quick or slow? His homeopathic doctor found it awfully slow. He is married to his girlfriend now, and his mother came to their wedding.

In the last followup, 16 months after I first saw him, he feels fine, and all the symptoms are gone. His job is fine. He is at peace with his wife and talks about his job; he made up a new schedule so everybody could have a lunch break. What does he like to eat? "Sometimes we like to go out to have dinner. My wife is a very good cook."

Did you experience the change in his miasmatic situation? Perhaps later we'll see another layer, but we dealt with the psoric and the tubercular miasms. I think those are finished.

Hahnemann says that after prescribing the remedies for the miasms, you come back to latent psora, and then the patient will be fine.

The psora in him was active again after the tubercular miasm, and now he is in latent psora. This can go on for months or years. One year later, he had no problems.

Homeopaths are like the quiet cat watching for mice. Watch calmly and peacefully and observe, and only when there is a new picture, jump!

CHAPTER 5

Cancer and the Cancer Miasm

When the psoric, sycotic, syphilitic, and tubercular miasms are all present together in a person, the cancer miasm also may be present. The cancer miasm does not have to be there, but it may be. The other four miasms must be present for the cancer miasm to be present.

If all of the other four miasms are present and the patient's health is suppressed, the cancer miasm may show itself. When the first four are present together, there is also the possibility, though not the surety, of getting the disease of cancer. For example, if a child is not strong, has all four miasms present, and gets a vaccination or receives a similarly strong stress or trauma, she can develop the cancer disease at a very young age.

With regard to cancer, remember that we are talking at times about the cancer miasm and at other times about the cancer disease. Just as with syphilis and tuberculosis, the cancer miasm has the same name as the disease that spawned it.

The concept of a "cancer miasm" is still very young—only 50 to 60 years old—and is attributed to the Scottish physician Donald MacDonald Foubister (1902–1988), who worked at the London Homeopathic Hospital and was a fellow of the Faculty of Homoeopathy as well as its president and dean. He wrote:

> "My interest in Carcinosin was aroused by a chance experience: that of having in the outpatient department, simultaneously, two children born of mothers who were, during the pregnancy, suffering from cancer of the breast. These children presented a remarkably similar appearance, having blue sclerotics, a cafe au lait complexion, and numerous moles. Both children suffered from insomnia. I had previously been given a therapeutic hint that where there was a family history of cancer, Carcinosin sometimes cured insomnia, and had used it occasionally in insomnia with success.
>
> "I wondered if one could regard these children, having been nourished by cancerous blood, as exhibiting these characteristics on

account of the mother's condition, in other words, was this a sort of proving of Carcinosin, or was it a coincidence.

"The immediate course open was to study the antecedents of children with that appearance to find out whether this appearance was associated with a strong family history of cancer or not. In the outpatient department we began by checking the family history and giving Carcinosin to children with that appearance. During the first few years detailed notes [were] taken by one of my clinical assistants of 200 cases in which we had tested the remedy with or without success. Gradually the picture of Carcinosin emerged.

"It soon became apparent that children of what we came to regard as [having] the 'Carcinosin appearance' did not show the kind of family history we had almost expected to find. In many instances there was a strong family history of cancer, but in others there was a strong family history of tuberculosis, of diabetes and pernicious anaemia, or a combination of all these more strongly represented than in the average family; only occasionally there was no such history. It would, of course, require a great deal of research to prove this.

"Gradually we gained the impression that in addition to the "Carcinosin appearance" and a tendency to insomnia, even in young children, there was a tendency to have an inflammatory illness, usually whooping cough or pneumonia, very early in life, and therefore almost always severely. For instance, whooping cough at five months fits into the Carcinosin picture. If, for the sake of argument, we accept McDonagh's concept that there are two basic diseases, inflammation and tumour formation, also the teaching of Rudolph Steiner, then it might not be too far fetched to regard this tendency to inflammation as a reaction against inherited tendencies." (Foubister, Donald M. "The Carcinosin Drug Picture." Bombay, India: Homeopathic Medical Publishers, 1958.)

Thus the idea of familial cancer traits was born. Dr. Foubister observed that these children were very **sensitive and small**. He wrote down what he observed and wondered about it. He reasoned that perhaps patients who presented with these symptoms could be prevented from developing cancer by treating them with a remedy made from a woman's breast cancer. In some cases, it helped.

Through the years, it became clear to Dr. Foubister that if a child had these symptoms—**weakness, sensitivity, sleeplessness, crying all night, blue sclera, and café au lait spots on the skin**—the child could be helped with *Carcinosin*, a nosode made from cancerous tissue. The child did not have to be born of a mother with cancer; he only had to have the symptoms. This new pattern of symptoms, beyond other known patterns, led to the understanding of the cancer miasm as a unique energetic pattern of illness.

There are many ideas as to the causes or origins of the disease of cancer. In general, many believe that the disease of cancer is the result of some form of suppression—perhaps a profound idea, when we consider how many ways we can be suppressed—not the least of which is suppression by medical treatments.

There are consequences to vaccinating a child against a specific disease. These vaccinations take away the possibility for the child to react from his inner self to the surface—to discharge something from the inside and bring it to the outside. I have observed in little children that under normal circumstances, when there is no interference, the newborn child of about five to six weeks of age will show a skin eruption (mostly on the neck, a little behind the ears, and a little on the face.) The psora is coming out. Another infant will develop a fiery red diaper rash—a little sycosis coming to the surface. Loving mothers, disturbed by the appearance of skin problems or fearful that something is wrong, treat the skin eruptions with zinc baby cream (given away free in some maternity hospitals). This is the first suppression. They're suppressing, not realizing what they are doing.

Children need these discharges and diseases to rid themselves of the miasmatic influences with which they are born—and we are all born with miasmatic influence. When a baby is born of psoric parents and her body tries to get rid of psora, she will itch. If she is born with sycosis, she will get inflammations.

In addition to the more general skin rashes, children's diseases—chickenpox, measles, and mumps—can be wonderfully helpful as vehicles for transporting problems and disturbances from the inside to the outside.

Skin eruptions are one such powerful vehicle, ridding the organism of the deeper problems before they are given time to worsen. These skin eruptions come and go from the upper body to the lower body and disappear in the most natural way possible. If, during a childhood disease, the skin eruption goes from the hands or feet up to the center, eventually there may be problems such as pneumonia after the measles. The cases I have seen reacting in this way were vaccinated cases. Never does a spontaneous old-fashioned measles or mumps progress in this way, and I have never seen this in children who are treated homeopathically. It is best to let these children's diseases come out!

A child's reactions to vaccination will help show to what miasm he belongs. A cancer miasm reaction would be similar to a psoric reaction—it would have weakness, malaise, and a lack of reaction.

Cancer Miasm vs. Cancer Disease

People with any miasmatic state can get the disease of cancer. The cancer miasm does not have to be on top; it just has to be a part of the miasmatic influence in the person. For example, one person may feel fine, then starts to talk about pain in his abdomen, and six weeks later is dead. Another patient may have been living with cancer for 20 years. Both cancers are malignant, but the difference lies in how the cancer manifests, how the person is in the cancer. How the cancer affects the person depends on what is in the "miasm pot" of the patient.

When cancer spreads quickly after the onset of some little pain, as in the first example above, this indicates that a hidden illness was destroying the tissue of the liver and the pancreas, and it was happening quickly. The destruction and hiding of the syphilitic miasm plus the rapid growth of the sycotic miasm were there.

If a patient with a brain tumor comes for a homeopathic consultation after having had it for 10 years, she is certainly psoric. This kind of tumor is slow, often benign, because it is not growing through the tissue. One can live a long time with a psoric tumor.

The origin of any disease state belongs to the underlying miasm(s), but the outcome of having any particular miasm does not have to result in any specific disease. It is important to make this distinction.

I want to be very clear about the difference between treating the disease and treating the miasm and when to use the nosode. Our allopathic backgrounds make us a little lazy. We often mistakenly think, "Cancer disease requires *Carcinosin*," or "Tuberculosis disease requires *Tuberculinum*." A patient can have the disease of cancer without having the cancer miasm dominant. It is important to understand this point.

A psoric patient with cancer can be helped, even cured, with a psoric remedy, such as Calcarea carbonica, if her state is psoric and her symptoms belong to Calcarea carbonica, even when there are tissue changes.

In the same way, not everyone who has the cancer miasm dominant will have the disease of cancer. It is possible that there is no specific incidence of cancer (disease) in the family history. Still, when we see the state and the symptoms of the cancer miasm, we need to give a remedy that covers the cancer miasm (not only *Carcinosin*). We know that when we see evidence of the cancer miasm as well as sycotic, syphilitic, and tubercular influences in the patient, it is possible for that person to develop the disease of cancer. The dominant presence of the cancer miasm is not required for the patient to develop cancer. However, a patient with symptoms pointing to four miasms who receives a strong negative influence—suppression, stress, or trauma—is in a state where she can develop the cancer disease. I want to stress this point and make it very clear because this thinking applies to all the miasms we have studied and all the diseases we will see.

We think about diseases as belonging to different miasms, but as homeopaths, we are not treating the disease; we are treating the state. Only this brings cure.

If somebody with the cancer miasm develops a headache and needs to dance to make himself feel better, he may need *Carcinosin* to rid himself of his headache even though he does not have the disease of cancer. When somebody with the cancer miasm lies in her bed with the disease of cancer, has hard knots in her chest or glands, says she does not need homeopathic treatment, yet says, "I will make my will," she might need *Conium*. We would not give *Carcinosin* just because she has cancer.

Mental and Emotional Symptoms and Expressions of the Cancer Miasm

Compassion for animals and people
Love of dancing
Extremely sensitive to nature, beauty, classical music
Loves lightning and thunderstorms
Loves nature
Disturbances have no way out—no outlets
Perfectionism
Refinement
Romantic feelings and ideas
Sacrifices his desires
Suppresses his feelings
Sensitive to feelings of others

The cancer miasm has psoric, sycotic, and syphilitic symptoms, with the addition of some typical tubercular symptoms such as love of travel and respiratory symptoms. As with all miasms, the cancer miasm has its own unique characteristic behaviors and symptoms.

Cancer will suppress his own feelings to avoid hurting others, and because of this, he may withdraw. While syphilis will withdraw because he does not feel kindly or nice toward others and wants to cover it up, cancer will hide (a piece of syphilis in him) because he is sensitive to hurting someone else's feelings. Cancer people are **caring**, **loving**, **unselfish** people who are easy to get along with—maybe too easy. We sometimes see this even in small children. Some do not like to express things because Mom might be hurt when she hears it. Others will say, "I cannot tell my friend something because it might hurt her." There is a lot of holding back. When someone holds back, **suppressing himself** and his feelings for his entire life because he might hurt someone else, he can get the disease of cancer. If he keeps everything inside and has no outlets, he can get the disease of cancer. Of course, there are other reasons—for example, cancer due to environmental agents, including smoking, or passive smoking and toxic workplace situations.

If cancer has hurts of her own, she does not ask for help. For example, *Carcinosin* will not speak about her problems to other people. She behaves a lot like *Staphysagria*, keeping things inside. She is so sweet and sensitive that she can be **easily hurt and abused**. She suffers from things and does not react outwardly until she gets a remedy; until then, her energy cannot come out. Cancer takes many things in but cannot repel them or throw them off. She voluntarily suppresses her feelings. She tries to work things out in a nice way, which may be nice for other people, but it is not nice for her because it can kill her.

Cancer has opinions about things, but she never tells other people what to do or how to behave. She is **not bossy or pushy** with others. She is not showy. She puts herself in the background. She **allows herself to be dominated**. Cancer is too refined and sensitive to push others around and generally keeps silent.

The cancer miasm has a desire to care for people. He feels pity for others and wants to help others. He will **sacrifice himself for other people**. Social work is a job that suits him. But he cares in such an extreme way that he becomes overwhelmed and burned out and cannot care anymore.

The cancer miasm is very sensitive. She is **sensitive to people, animals, beauty, nature—everything**. She loves romance. She is sensitive like tuberculosis but reacts differently. For example, cancer may **cry sentimentally** about the beautiful purple sky and remember it forever and ever because nature is so beautiful. She is easily astonished and may cry easily at beautiful things. Weeping from music belongs to both the tubercular and cancer miasms. I cannot imagine *Carcinosin* listening to music without a beautiful melody. The rhythm of drums is intolerable to *Carcinosin*. She likes **classical music**—beautiful, peaceful music.

The cancer miasm **loves to dance**. He likes refined music and refined dancing. Even though he may be tired, he feels better from dancing. The tubercular person's energy goes up and down in sharp spikes—first the kicks and then the exhaustion. The energy of cancer also rises and falls but not in such spikes; it is more of a slightly wavy line up and down from the baseline.

Cancer loves nature. She loves to see animals in their natural environments. She enjoys lightning and thunderstorms. She experiences these events as beautiful.

Cancer sometimes likes things that people in the other miasms fear. Cancer has a **great love of animals**, in all ways. He may spend all of his money to save animals. He may leave all his money to his animals or buy a cemetery plot and build a statue for his pet. Sensitivity to animals expressed in these extreme ways is part of cancer. In courts of law, judges and lawyers sometimes get involved in divorces to make arrangements for the dog—one week with the husband, one week with the wife. This seems to go beyond reasonable limits, but this is how cancer can show concern for animals. Some of my patients come into the consulting room with a dog or cat and tell me they cannot leave their pets alone for even a few minutes until we're finished with the consultation. This is appropriate behavior for mothers with babies but more care than is necessary with pets. Sometimes people who cannot express their feelings toward other people overdo with too much compassion for animals. We see this strong feeling toward animals in *Carcinosin* and some other small remedies. But *Carcinosin* does not undervalue people like some other remedies that have extreme love for animals. Rather *Carcinosin* shares his concern for both people *and* animals.

The cancer miasm loves the sea air. He likes to be in the sun. He loves the feeling and the **beauty of the sea**, the sun coming up, white foam on the waves. Tuberculosis loves being in the mountains. Cancer will go to the mountains as well, but she likes to be there because it is pristine and beautiful.

> *Go on holiday to the mountains and bring psora, sycosis, tuberculosis, and cancer (syphilis will go by himself). They all love a trip to the mountains, but each behaves differently. Sycosis will be the first to reach the top, and he shouts and dances. Tuberculosis will run to see what is over the next ridge. Cancer will be quiet—"Ah, it's so beautiful." Psora will finally catch up, huffing and puffing.*

Like tuberculosis, cancer **loves to travel**. Tuberculosis needs the change and excitement that travel provides. Cancer may take an art tour to Italy to see the beautiful art museums and old churches; he really appreciates beauty. Cancer wants to experience the beauty of the world and to connect with other people. He is very social, while tuberculosis is more egotistical.

Cancer is a **perfectionist**. She gets this from psora. She can be meticulous and fastidious but not like *Arsenicum*, doing fussy, useless things for no good reason. Cancer's fastidiousness is about **beauty**. Her clothing and home may not be spotlessly clean, but her clothes and her environment must have a perfect combination of colors. The paintings must go with the tapestries, the drapes with the carpets—her interests and abilities are creative and artistic.

Love of **chocolate** is well known in the cancer miasm. In the supermarket, cancer may have a meticulous list of everything he needs—a perfect list—with chocolate at the top. There are several types and a variety of tastes in chocolate—sweet, light-brown milk chocolate; plain or with a creamy filling; dark, bitter chocolate. The people who love plain milk chocolate belong mostly to remedies like *Sulphur* (desire for sweetness). Those who love chocolate with the creamy insides belong mostly to remedies like *Calcarea carbonica* (desire for creamy things). Remedies like *Sepia, Natrum muriaticum,* and *Carcinosin* prefer dark, bitter chocolate. We would never give our patients a remedy based on the desire for one type of chocolate, but understanding the difference in taste and the intensity behind the craving is helpful.

General and Physical Symptoms of the Cancer Miasm

- Absence of childhood diseases
- Blue sclera
- Café au lait spots
- Childhood diseases as an adult
- Incorrect disease patterns
- Mononucleosis
- Pernicious anemia
- Presence of or influence of the other four miasms
- No outlets—stress goes inward to physical disease
- Tumors

The cancer miasm may be present in a patient when there is a family history of cancer or diabetes or when the patient's presenting disease pattern is unusual or abnormal. For example, people should get children's diseases when they are children, which is the normal pattern. Getting chickenpox or any other children's disease as an adult or having them again as an adult belongs to the cancer miasm. Another characteristic belonging to the cancer miasm is the nonoccurrence of children's diseases. Those who are exposed to other children and do not contract children's diseases, or those children who contract the disease shortly after birth or as very young infants, are expressing the cancer miasm. When a young child has an adult disease, this is an expression of the cancer miasm. With the cancer miasm, something about the **disease pattern** may be wrong.

The cancer miasm manifests the aggressiveness of the tubercular miasm and the destructiveness of the syphilitic miasm in the physical body. The person is not necessarily aggressive or destructive, but many of the person's physical diseases are aggressive and break down the body.

Mononucleosis belongs to the cancer miasm. Most, but not all mononucleosis happens during puberty and the teenage years. Sometimes, after **mononucleosis**, the patient gets chronic fatigue. She can become exhausted, unable to do things for years. She remains in a weak, infectious state, with perhaps a little fever. Sometimes glands are swollen. This patient has the cancer miasm.

Another clinical sign of the cancer miasm, strongly linked with the syphilitic miasm, is ulcerative colitis. This condition, in reality, may develop into the disease of cancer.

Clinically, diseases such as pernicious anemia are linked to the cancer miasm—wasting away, not being able to build oneself up. There is significant damage to the blood, which shows the influence of the syphilitic miasm.

Nephrotic syndrome is the result of a combination of the miasms. It is almost as deep as cancer. It is very difficult to treat because there is a malfunctioning of the kidney tissue indicating that destruction in the kidneys has occurred. Diabetes in the patient or in the family history is a sign of the cancer miasm. Characteristic visual signs of the cancer miasm are blue sclera, café au lait spots on the skin, and, of course, tumors.

Cancer Remedies

Carcinosin and *Scirrhinum* are two of the cancer miasm nosodes. The cancer nosodes were made from tissue taken from different cancer sites in the body—intestinal, lung, and breast—as well as from different types of cancers. In *Kent's Repertory* there is a list of cancer remedies, each of which, if understood deeply, can guide us in understanding and in differentiating both the disease of cancer and the various aspects and presentations of the cancer miasm.

View *Kent's* rubric: **GENERALITIES; CANCEROUS** *affections* (49). The remedies listed in *Kent's Repertory* in bold type are some of the remedies that are known to cure cancer: *Arsenicum album, Bromium, Carbo animalis, Conium, Lycopodium, Nitric acid, Phosphorus, Phytolacca,* and *Silica. Carcinosin* is not listed in *Kent's Repertory* because the remedy did not yet exist. *Radium bromatum* and the other radiums are also important in the treatment of the cancer miasm as well as in the disease of cancer. Again, remember that in treating homeopathically, cancer, the disease, is part of a more complex disease state, and we must differentiate the state of the patient, not merely the disease.

It is good to look at some of the rubrics for tumors from *Kent's Repertory*:

- GENERALITIES; TUMORS, *cystic* (11): agar., apis., **Bar-c.**, *brom., calc., calc.s.,* **Graph.**, hep., nit.ac., sil., sulph.
- GENERALITIES; TUMORS, *cystic; atheroma* (1): bar-c.
- GENERALITIES; TUMORS, *cystic; cheloid* (1): sil.
- GENERALITIES; TUMORS, *cystic; erectile* (4): *lyc., nit-ac., phos.,* staph.
- GENERALITIES; TUMORS, *cystic; fibroid* (6): *calc.,* **Calc-f.**, *calc-s., con.,* **Phos.**, **Sil.**
- GENERALITIES; TUMORS, *cystic; neuroma* (2): calc., staph.
- GENERALITIES; TUMORS, *cystic; sarcoma* (2): bar-c., calc-f.
- GENERALITIES; TUMORS, *cystic; steatoma, suppurating* (2): *calc., carb-v.*
- GENERALITIES; TUMORS, *ccystic;* r*eappearing every 4 weeks* (1): *calc.*

Today, we often use the words "tumor" and "cancer" interchangeably, as if they mean the same thing. In Kent's time, a tumor was a lump that did not move under pressure but was not necessarily cancerous. In his time, cancer referred to a certain change in the tissue that was shown by a biopsy. Be aware of the difference in clinical expressions between now and then. If we tell someone in today's clinic that he has a tumor, his first thought may be that he has cancer. When we use the word "cancer" today, we think of something that is almost incurable. In former times, perhaps homeopaths treated many patients with undetected cancer. Without knowing that their patient had a cancer, under homeopathic treatment, if the patient became well, the cancer was also unknowingly cured.

A patient's appearance may indicate that he has the disease of cancer, for example, wasting, grayness, and hollow eyes. Today, modern equipment can often find hidden tumors, even though they are tiny. In Kent's time, however, he saw only things like vision loss, rectal bleeding, or the feel of the tumor.

The picture of the cancer miasm is very similar to the picture of *Carcinosin,* but treatment of the cancer miasm does not automatically call for *Carcinosin.* There are many remedies that successfully treat the cancer miasm. To find the best remedy, we must look for the strange, rare, and peculiar symptoms in a patient, including the symptoms of the miasm.

Some of the symptoms of the nosode *Carcinosin* are:

- Fastidious, perfectionism
- Sensitive to surroundings, music, beauty, nature
- Sympathy and anxiety for others
- Strong sense of duty and responsibility
- Love of animals
- Love of dancing, better from dancing even though weak
- Love of chocolate
- Feels good near the sea—walking on the beach, swimming, sailing
- Love of thunderstorms
- Chronic or prolonged insomnia

Sometimes we come up against a barrier in the course of treating our patients. Whatever potency we use, the remedy cannot seem to go "over" or "through" the wall. Just as the tubercular nosode, if called for, can unblock a tubercular case, if the symptoms of the patient fit the picture, the *Carcinosin* nosode can remove the block in the energy of the vital force and the patient can improve.

Treating the Disease of Cancer

If we can find the constitutional remedy, the simillimum, it is possible to cure some patients of cancer. If we cannot initially find the simillimum, perhaps a well-chosen remedy can give them the needed time for their vital force to create a better state, where the simillimum can be more easily discovered.

Although we see some cancer patients in our practice, most go to the oncology clinic or the hospital. If they receive chemotherapy, these powerful drugs kill almost every possibility for the vital force to react with symptoms. When the patient cannot produce vital symptoms, the homeopath has nothing on which to prescribe. Even when we know a patient's state, it's difficult for a remedy to strengthen that person if she is taking chemotherapy. Most do not survive for long.

To find the state of the patient, we have to hope that the vital force is still active enough to show its state, and then we must find the characteristic symptoms of the patient. It is best to go back to the time just before the cancer, particularly before there was any treatment for the cancer, and find the characteristics and the modalities of that state.

If we find the state that existed before the cancer and the patient receives the correct remedy, there are two possible results. The vital force of the patient is either strong enough to bring her back to a healthier state or not strong enough, so that all we can do is palliate her pain and make her more comfortable. Sometimes we have to find the constitutional remedy with the help of the family. Someone with a brain tumor may not be able to tell us how he was before the tumor.

Treating cancer is sometimes like trying to treat a person who is very old. By this, I mean that the organism is no longer showing personal, characteristic symptoms. When we see a person with a strong vitality at 30 years of age, the personal symptoms spill out in the first consultation. When we see a person who is 84 years old, we may hear about some pain in the shoulder and maybe some sleeplessness. We have to go all the way back to the patient's youth, childhood, sometimes even to infancy, to get some useful symptoms—and she does not remember! These symptoms are gone for her. Of course, there are some "young" 80-year-olds who can go back to a time when they were hurt and tell us about it. And they can give their food desires and strong characteristic symptoms, though this is not usual. But when a patient of 45 years of age is near death with cancer and has been treated allopathically, we see in her the same "state" as in someone who is 92 years old, complaining of some pain in the shoulder and knee.

To find the correct remedy, we must be able to understand the personal symptoms, differentiate the patient's characteristics from the pathology of the disease, and then disregard all symptoms that belong only to the pathology, without distinguishing characteristics.

We can use modalities, generals, and mind symptoms, but finding these is not an easy task. We have to look for these with a magnifying glass, like Sherlock Holmes. If the modality we see is the result of allopathic treatment, we cannot use it.

We must look for the picture of the patient apart from the general conditions of the disease. For example, in a series of cancer patients with whom we may consult, all may fear that they only have a few months to live, all are probably receiving chemical therapy and/or radiation and have had x-rays, and many have a bald head as a result of the drug treatment. How do they react to these things? They all fear death because this is their reality. Try to differentiate by understanding how they reacted when they got the message. What did each do? One cried, one became pale, one got angry, another got diarrhea, another phoned his mother or father, another counted his money, and another began to arrange everything for the children's future. We must be as logical as we can when treating and prescribe on what the vital force is asking for with signs and symptoms. Thinking about the miasms helps us decipher what we see—helps us to be clearer in our understanding.

We must think about dosage somewhat differently when treating cancer patients because there is so much going on in the body at the physical level. With one higher dose of the remedy, the patient may feel better, but the illness may go on. We may have the initial impression that the remedy is working wonderfully, but the illness continues. Using lower potencies, the possibilities are better. We must follow the path of the disease as it changes rapidly.

In homeopathy, there are many fairy tales. One is that old symptoms always come back. This does not always happen.

Some homeopaths worry that if a patient had cancer in the past, the cancer will come back. If the patient did not die of his cancer 10 years ago and at this moment is given a homeopathic remedy, is he going to die from being given the correct homeopathic remedy now? If he did not die from allopathic treatment, why would he die from homeopathy?

In treating patients with the disease of cancer, we have to assess very carefully for improvement to determine whether we are turning the energy away from death and toward life. If the cancer disease is beyond the level of cure, the remedy's energy will be used up quickly. Cancer patients must be seen much more often if they are beyond the possibility of cure.

Homeopathy at the End of Life

In the end, we will all die of something. In former times, people died in the most natural way. They got tired of life, lay down, and did not live anymore. Many of our parents may have died in a natural way, lying down and telling their children goodbye. Dying is not the nicest thing we will experience in life, but it can be nicer than it is today.

I had treated a colleague for the last 20 years of her 30-year battle with cancer. She got much better. About three weeks before she died, she visited me in the consulting room. She told me she was feeling weak for the first time in her life, and she was coming to get a remedy to feel stronger. I spoke with her every day, and at a certain moment she realized her energy was going down. She asked me if there was a way for cure, and I said, "No. We are on the way to the end of your life." And she said, "So I have work to do." Sometimes she had pain, but the remedy relieved it immediately. I visited her one night, and she was on a bed surrounded by candles and flowers. She spoke about how well she had been feeling, how glad she was that she had had 20 extra years of good living, and how glad she was that she could know ahead of time that she was dying. She told me how nice it was to be able to divide her possessions and give her things to the people she cared about. Then she became too weak to talk.

I saw how homeopathy could help people die peacefully. I hope that everybody can die in a similar situation, surrounded by friends and flowers and feeling positive about saying good-bye.

As homeopaths, our first goal is to cure our patients, but if there is no possibility of cure, we have to help them meet their end in a positive and good way. People do not need to be drugged, unconscious and unprepared. That is what allopathy does now. Our hope is to help our patients die near their families, making things straight that went wrong, preparing for the end.

Cancer Case 1: Woman With Marriage Problems, Depression, and Anger

Video Presentation and Case Description

The following discussion was captured as it occurred during a video presentation and case description. Student questions and comments appear within brackets. "HH" indicates a question or comment by Henny Heudens, and "P" indicates "patient."

The remedy used in this case is well known by name but not well known by use. This lady is 43 years old. One of the problems she has is that her marriage is starting to break up. Her husband travels a lot and sees other women, and she knows this. It's the second marriage for both of them. They have a little girl, and she is their reason for remaining in the marriage. The daughter is now eight years old. There are a lot of fights and quarreling—often one parent stays upstairs, and one stays downstairs. They cannot communicate anymore.

In fact, the problem started between them with the birth of the child. The patient felt that her husband did not support her during the pregnancy or delivery. It was a difficult delivery; the child was too small and had problems and had to be placed in an incubator. The mother felt very tired and depressed. When the baby came home after a few weeks, she cried for six months. She could not be calmed down except for lying or sitting in the lap of the mother. This left no time for the husband anymore.

The patient tells me why her marriage is not a brilliant one. "He always leaves me alone. Not only does he not tell me about his job or share his feelings, but for the past six months I have had to take care of our daughter alone." Now that her child is eight years old, the situation is as bad as before, or worse. One to two days before her period, the patient experiences an outburst of feelings. This is an exacerbation of her feelings that have accumulated over the weeks and years. (Some call it premenstrual syndrome [PMS]).

The woman has a special behavior. In my consulting room, she said, "You know, you have to change your light. This is not healthy for you to be under this light all day." She said it in quite a nice way. She has the feeling she can foresee what will happen in the future. She has a swelling of the thyroid gland. She has dreams about the future. She dreams she would like to go away but is kept as a prisoner or held by someone's arms. When she and her husband do sleep in the same bed, she sleeps with the child between them because she feels so alone in the room. She sleeps superficially and awakens at the least noise. She is bored with her job and housework, so she began a career like her husband's; he is a traveling salesman. However, she does not want to travel until the child is older and can be left alone. "Then," she says, "my husband will not be able to be with other women."

When they have holidays she feels much better. They do not always share holidays, but the ones she shares with her husband and daughter are fine. For the holidays the husband takes alone, she goes on holiday with her child. She likes to be in nature—not alone with the child, but with people. She loves to be with people. When she found a picture of her second/current husband's lover in his suitcase, she took the picture, put it on her shelf, and during a quarrel, showed it to him and tore it up in front of him.

In her former marriage, she had two children. She felt the husband did not accept her pregnancy. He kicked her in her abdomen. She wanted to kick him back, but she did not do it because she knew he had no limits. If he were really mad, he might kill her and the child, then he'd be in prison and she would be dead. She resisted irritating him because of the children.

Her father died at 55 years of age of leukemia. She has the feeling she will not live to be old. Because her husband has outside relationships, she is very depressed. After the birth of this third child, she had the feeling that she did not want any more babies. She chose sterilization. Since that time, there isn't much anger anymore, but there is deep depression and some anger. She has menstrual periods with a lot of blood; she bleeds strongly for three days. The blood is black, then bright red, then black again. There is pain from the beginning until the end of the bleeding. She has pain in her back that goes into her thighs, with a feeling that her legs are stiff. She has an awful fear of being alone. She says she needs a hand to pull her out of her depression. She is very angry when she thinks about it.

P—My husband will exchange me for another woman. When I think of this, I really could kill him, but I won't do it.

HH—Is there anything that makes you happy?

P—Yes, mountains and snow. Swimming in the sea is wonderful. Animals—cats are so nice to cuddle.

Temperature? Spring is okay; winter is too cold for her. When her husband is downstairs, she weeps; when he is gone, she does not weep. She has a headache from her neck forward to the front of her head. She has been sexually active since the age of 15 years; at 16 years of age she might have had sex 6 to 10 times in one weekend.

When she was six weeks old, she had whooping cough. As a young child she had hepatitis. There were no difficult illnesses in her adult life. Before the consultation, I had a letter from her. (This is exceptional.) It was very specific and very neat. She wrote down all the symptoms she gave me later on, except the real history about her husband. On one of the pages, she wrote, "I have one goal in my life, and that is that a man loves me, cuddles me, and gives me what I need. I cannot give myself to anyone who does not do this for me. For what am I living? I weep and weep and weep. I have lost my control. In former times, I had this feeling only before menstruation, but now I have it all month long. I deserve so much attention and love, but I get the contrary."

This is contradictory. What are normal goals in life? When one has a goal such as this woman's, it means that if your husband dies or if he looks for another woman, your life is lost. Of course, we all know these are difficult things to suffer, but having as your only goal a husband who loves you implies that she has no self-confidence and relies on others to provide it. The excessive sex in her teens was about the same thing—love me, love me, love me. She is not that young anymore. She has life experience now, but she still feels that she has never been loved. If you feel loved, this would not be your life's goal.

Cancer Case 1—Analysis

How is she miasmatically? [*Depressed, wanting to kill her husband.*] Happily, her mind is not that ill. She is ill emotionally. Syphilitic patients may be physically deformed, or as with her, their emotions are deformed. This marriage is of a bad quality. She tells me I'm her last hope to give her back her feelings and restore her marriage. This is syphilitic because of the thoughts of killing, the black bleeding during menses, and leukemia in the family. What else is there? [*High sex drive.*] [*Sycosis.*]

How about her desire to be in nature with other people? If the sycotic miasm were strong in her, how would she be? Sycotic people want to be with other people in action—parties, dancing, and so forth. I once read in a newspaper that a Japanese boy died during a sexual act with three girls while in the sea—excessive sex at the seashore—*Medorrhinum.*

Why does she take a child of that age into her bed? Maybe to tell her husband she does not want to have sex with him anymore because of his cheating, perhaps for her own comfort. But we will not prescribe on theories. [*She has a swollen thyroid gland. She is hyperthyroid. This could be sycosis.*] [*Where are her first two children?*] They are grown, and she wanted to start a new family.

[*There is a strong lack of connection with the first family and husband, even with friends.*] Yes; the situation repeats itself in the second marriage; most of the time there is a reason why it happens again and again.

[*I find it strange that she wants so badly to be loved but left her first two children.*] If we can help her, we will see her husband sleeping with her again and her putting the child out of her bed.

What more can we say of this woman? She is not a bad woman. [*She needs a lot of support. I think she's a typical woman.*] In such a case, be aware of not going into it with your feelings. Be objective.

What are the needs of a healthy woman? [*To love and give love.*] What are the needs of a man? [*The same.*] Women also want to be respected. When a woman does not feel the need to be respected as a woman, she is ill.

As homeopaths, we must be able to recognize any expression of imbalance in each and every characteristic of our patients.

We know there is always a range of "normal/healthy" expression and when a patient has strong feelings, attitudes, or behaviors that are outside the norm for health, these expressions are as important to us as an irregular heartbeat or an elevated white blood count. When a woman today is ambitious, this is not especially unusual. Women are strong, women have power in the world, and a woman can be quite powerful while still retaining her femininity. But when she loses her more feminine feelings and outlook and adopts a more combative masculine way, these are signals that she is leaving the center of balance and moving toward imbalance. The same is true for men. There is a general range of what is healthy gender behavior. When I am in my consulting room with a man who is quite feminine in his behavior, I am alert to the possibility that something is out of balance. Be objective. Be unprejudiced. Many men feel suppressed by women of power—possibly a signal of stress or imbalance. Both sexes need love and attention, but in different ways. That a woman cares for her child is totally normal. If she takes her healthy child in the bed to separate herself from her husband, this indicates an imbalance. That a woman can leave her children because she prefers to start a new life shows illness in the emotional sphere.

Why does someone start a new life? If there were mistakes and instead of working through the problems and learning from my mistakes, I choose to leave the situation to avoid being reminded of it, it's likely that I will make the same mistakes again. I'm sure she did this with the best of intentions, yet this woman's history is one of making mistakes, turning the page, and trying to start over—but taking the illness with her. The rucksack, filled with all of life's experiences, travels with a person.

What miasms are in this patient's case?

- *Syphilis*: Sending her children away, having the desire to kill, feeling revengeful anger, experiencing a lack of connection
- *Sycosis*: Excessive sexual behavior as a teenager
- *Psora*: Very cold and weak, needs to be loved to the point of making it her goal, feeling forsaken, lacking something sufficient in her structure
- *Tuberculosis*: Love of mountains, desire to start new things, whooping cough when very young

What are the positive things about this woman? [*She did not immediately hit her husband back; she's concerned for her children.*] [*She spent the first six months with that baby on her lap.*] Yes, this was healthy. The baby needed this.

How about her behavior with other people? Her first comment was showing concern for my health (the light in my office). Do we hear any problems with other people? She wants to be together with people in nature.

What miasm is this woman? Cancer. What is the remedy? *Carcinosin.* We see all the miasms and the combination of being a loving person to nature, animals, and other people. This is a wonderful example of *Carcinosin.* The rubrics I used for her were:

- Anxious about others
- Sympathetic
- Desire to travel
- Love for animals
- Love of nature
- Fear of being alone
- Clairvoyance

Let's look at a few of the remedies in the rubric "MIND, CLAIRVOYANCE" in *Kent's Repertory*:

- *Aconite* knows the time he will die (psoric).
- *Anacardium* hears voices that are telling him what to do (syphilitic).
- *Arnica* has out-of-body feelings.

Out-of-body experiences—looking down and seeing your body as if you are separate from your body—is syphilitic because there is a separation from the self. If you look carefully at the remedies in this rubric, you will find several that experience "after-death" symptoms. There are remedies that hear voices, singing, or bells ringing. Under "MIND, DELUSIONS" in the repertories, we find all of those experiences. What does it mean for a person to be clairvoyant? [*They can go beyond that border that separates us from the paranormal.*] [*They sense things other people cannot sense.*] Yes; is this healthy? Your answer may depend on your own vision or experience, but try to be objective. [*Having the experience of clairvoyance always affects their lives.*] Yes; otherwise they would not tell about these experiences in their consult.

Is being clairvoyant healthy? Again, there are certain ranges of possibilities, which we can experience with our eyes and ears and with our minds. Having the ability to know more than you have to know is a kind of oversensitivity, and oversensitivity is illness. Even when people use their hypersensitivity for nice things, their lives can be ruined. They are often living at the edge of their limits. Think objectively about this to help your patients. Think about what they tell you. For example, they may see things behind them or have an angel who smiles at them. It is a "deformity" in their feelings. This is syphilitic.

All of the rubrics we talked about are rubrics that lead us to *Carcinosin.* Some of her other symptoms are:

- Desires salt, rich cream, licorice, cooked eggs
- Averse to fat
- The need to vomit immediately
- Likes cold drinks
- Needs coffee to be awake
- Likes to walk on the beach, cycle, play tennis
- Likes the open air
- Feels best in or on the water (sailing or swimming)

[*Did you like her?*] I was concerned about her. Did I like her? I did not have a feeling of liking her or not. Her face was very gray, not healthy. You can imagine the remedies she was given. *Sepia*—quite a good idea; *Phosphorus*—perhaps for the ice cream, although not enough on which to prescribe; and *Lycopodium*—hepatitis as a small child, lack of self-confidence, bossy, and dictatorial. None of the remedies worked.

How is the love for animals in *Nuphar luteum*? [*Exclusive.*] How is it in her? [*She cuddles her cats.*] Love for cats and animals is totally normal. But if you send away your children, do not feel love for your husband, and need to cuddle your cats, this is strange. How did the husband behave at the birth of their child? He did not support her in giving birth. What does this mean? Her report was that she had the feeling that he did not support her, but he never actually left. She felt he wasn't taking care of her. What is going on when a child is in the incubator and is happy only in the lap of the mother? The woman was disturbed emotionally; she could not feel support or love, just as she could not feel love for her first two children whom she sent to live with her former husband. Then she starts to cuddle the cat—a substitute for people.

As homeopaths, we do not have the luxury of taking what we observe in our patients for granted. We must be keen in our observation and keen in our understanding of the smallest detail to discern what is important to each case.

Imagine a nice family picture: two children, husband, and wife. It's time to get up, time to set the breakfast table. Mom is looking for the cat. The children are waiting for breakfast, and the mother is looking for the cat. Mom finds the cat and fusses over it but forgets about the children. This is unusual. She cannot give love to the children but gets love from the cats. Something in her feelings is not connected. *Carcinosin* has love for animals: They do things with animals that they cannot do with other people. What other remedies love animals? [*Natrum muriaticum, because they are withdrawn from people, but not as extreme as Nuphar luteum.*]

We gave her *Carcinosin*. In her history, her father died of leukemia, she has ailments from domination, and she had whooping cough at six weeks of age. *Carcinosin* is a remedy that has two possibilities in connection to children's diseases. You will see either no children's diseases at all when young or children's diseases in very young children shortly after birth. The time to get childhood diseases is when children start to go to school or preschool and are in contact with other children. Then they need diseases to protect themselves, to get their immune systems working. Whooping cough at six weeks of age is extraordinary, and in allopathic thinking, the baby's life is in danger. [*She also had hepatitis at a very young age.*] Even in the allopathic way of thinking, it shows how weak her vital force is. The cancer miasm also may include patients who get children's diseases as adults. [*Does this include patients who get chicken pox or mumps again as an adult?*] Yes—you should get these illnesses as a child, and if you do not or if you get them again as an adult, then this belongs to the cancer miasm.

Other keynotes of *Carcinosin* in this woman are:

- Fastidious (the letter she sent, noticing the light above me)
- Precocity—caring and responsible for others, thinking about others more than herself
- Loves chocolate
- Loves the sea, the beauty of the sun coming up, the white foam on the waves, the feeling of the sea (sycosis loves the waves and excitement of the sea)

Carcinosin hasn't a strong sense of fear. They have fear for the well-being of things in nature, concern for their surroundings, and fear that harm will come to the environment but not enough concern for themselves.

Cancer Case 1—Followup

Remember that I received this woman's letter before our appointment. She told me that she had an appointment on Friday the 13th but that I could read this beforehand so she would not have to take so much of my time. (She was considering me and disregarding herself—a *Carcinosin* expression.) After the remedy (about three weeks later), she was thinking about her husband and how their relationship had been changed by the child they both loved most—their daughter. She knew that she loved the child, and thought of the child as a gift from her husband. However, she did not feel happy after the difficult birth. Why was she not able to enjoy the child? Only because she felt bad during the birth. Was focusing on her difficult birth experience worth spoiling her life? She loved her husband before the birth, and he loved her. Why did her feelings change so dramatically during the birth?

Four months later she wrote, "Thanks. I did not know my health could be changed so dramatically."

After the remedy, she said, "I had the feeling my husband and I had to talk about what happened." She felt she had to tell him he gave her a wonderful girl. They thanked each other, and they started to talk. Since then, things have been changing. The patient told me, "I feel better with my menses. We had sexual contact some weeks ago. He told me he loved me, and he needed somebody to give him love. We have found each other again. It's not heaven, but it's not hell anymore."

What did the remedy do? This is a wonderful *Carcinosin* way to express feelings. She saw the child as a present her husband gave her. Over the years since, I have seen her from time to time. She always tells me how wonderful homeopathy is. She has only little problems now. This is a typical *Carcinosin* presentation, and her response shows the refinement of *Carcinosin.*

CHAPTER 6

OTHER MIASMS EMERGING

The more the miasms become combined in our patients, the more aggressive diseases become. In the disease of acquired immune deficiency syndrome (AIDS), there are symptoms from all five miasms. The more we suppress strong diseases such as gonorrhea, syphilis, tuberculosis, or cancer, the more dangerous the miasm that comes afterward.

Consider the pathology of the disease of AIDS. When the immune system and its ability to ward off the body's illnesses are suppressed, opposed, or circumvented by strong medicines, the body goes "on strike," so to speak. We could say that the vital force gives up trying to overcome "management"—it can no longer fight and stops working. In the past 50 years, antibiotics and strong drugs for nonspecific venereal diseases have been widely used to suppress the symptoms of gonorrhea and syphilis. When the tubercular way of life is added to this mix—for example, enjoyment from excitement and changing sexual partners—it is not strange that a disease such as AIDS can emerge. Society creates the soil for it. There is a pattern: Each time a new disease or miasm emerges, it is more lethal than its predecessors—killing people more surely than before.

With AIDS, there may be no escape, no way to reverse its effect. There are new drugs that increase T-cell levels, but these drugs similarly result in suppression as do vaccinations, penicillin, and steroids. When first discovered, these drugs were thought to cure. Now we know that although symptoms may abate with the use of these drugs, people become more ill than before. The future holds the answer. Homeopathically, when the human immunodeficiency virus (HIV)—the virus that is thought to cause AIDS—is suppressed, deeper diseases result.

Since disease is the result of a disturbance in energy, an illness establishes itself long before, and on a much deeper level, than its physical manifestations.

Using allopathic drugs can suppress and even transform or transmute the symptoms, but the nature of the disturbance remains and will disturb the physical level again. Only by touching the disturbance in the correct way on the energetic level can the energy right itself. By "killing" the symptoms of the disease, the vital force is pressed to bring out another disease to show the internal imbalance. Only by quieting the miasm—bringing it to its latent state—can the patient be cured.

This is what the old masters have taught us—**miasms spread**: psora by touch and syphilis and gonorrhea by sexual contact. The venereal diseases themselves, of course, spread by infecting new sexual partners. But beyond the transfer of the disease itself, the deeper illness, the miasmatic illness, can be transferred to a person's sexual partner. As we said earlier, if a healthy woman has sex with her husband and there is suppressed gonorrhea in his history, she can develop pain in the abdomen, menstrual problems, or a vaginal discharge. The medical books tell us that a woman who has *not* been exposed to venereal disease can develop "venereal ulcers" on the vulva. They are called venereal ulcers because they resemble the chancre. With our homeopathic miasmatic understanding, we now see how this can occur. She will not be diagnosed with gonorrhea or syphilis. Nevertheless, she is ill.

Some ask whether AIDS will be the next miasm. Keep in mind that we are theorizing now. We will have to wait and observe to see what happens. However, as with all the other miasms, the birth of an AIDS miasm is probable. Researchers and drug development teams are trying to cure AIDS, and some say they are getting results. Imagine that a drug treatment is found that can stop the AIDS virus from killing its victims and that these patients with AIDS begin to feel okay, with no clinical evidence of their disease. If these patients then have children, these babies could be born with no positive signs of active AIDS, yet be unable to recover from simple illnesses. Perhaps this will be the beginning of the AIDS miasm. Historically, the other five miasms developed in this fashion.

The future also may hold other influences that develop into miasms, bringing with them certain patterns in newborn children. Some homeopaths now refer to a cannabis miasm, and to my astonishment, they give their patients *Cannabis* simply because they or their parents have smoked pot. This is neither correct thinking nor the correct treatment of a miasm. This is isopathy. People must be treated according to their characteristic symptoms, adding the miasmatic analysis to our thinking.

It is incorrect to think that we should give everyone who has been exposed to a disease or a miasmatic influence the nosode of the disease or the miasm.

This is not the point of our discussion. It is isopathic prescribing to give *Tuberculinum* because the patient has tuberculosis or because he is tubercular. Perhaps *Cannabis* is a new miasm. If so, we will have to study its special collection of symptoms carefully to include them in a miasmatic analysis. We then must search the Materia Medica for the remedies with those predominant symptoms and use those remedies to cure.

Using Knowledge of the Miasms

Knowledge of miasms helps us choose the best remedy for our patients from the correct group of remedies. For example, for good health we need good water and good food from all the food groups: grains, dairy, meats, fruits, and vegetables. To eat correctly, we have to know how to recognize the characteristics of each food group and know which food belongs to which group. If we don't know that milk, butter, cheese, and cottage cheese belong to the dairy group and that asparagus and Brussels sprouts do not, we could make the wrong choices. To select the best remedy for the patient, we must recognize the miasms to know whether the patient's state shows psora, syphilis, sycosis, tuberculosis, or cancer and then select, from the correct group, a remedy that best covers the symptoms.

There are logical reasons for most illnesses, and when I cannot find the reason, I have trouble finding the remedy. For me, the vital force is a logical thing.

If we can discover the logic of how the vital force is working in a patient, we can find a solution. If we can see how all of the signs and symptoms relate to one another, it helps us see the miasm and choose the correct remedy. The same outward behavior or clinical disease can point to different miasms because they can manifest differently. We must always consider how the vital force is reacting. What are the symptoms expressing? This is the challenge with homeopathy. In difficult cases, miasmatic knowledge has helped me understand the patient and find the remedy. For years, I have taken the miasms out of the corners, and now they are in the middle of my mind. I am very aware of the signs and symptoms of the miasms as they present in patients.

The previous five chapters have presented a picture of the basic miasms. We know that syphilis and sycosis do not exist alone; they are mixed with psora. When we study the first three miasms well, we will better understand the mixture of symptoms in the tubercular and cancer miasms.

Miasms Seen Metaphorically

One of my students suggested a simple way to explain the combining of miasms within one patient: The miasms color everything that lies above. For example, if sycosis were yellow, with *Nux vomica* on top of it (let's say *Nux vomica* is some shade of blue), the picture we see would be some shade of green. We learn our remedies as individual colors, but the miasms underneath alter the colors on top. Therefore, sometimes we don't recognize the remedy. Think of a patient with more than one miasm as a series of photographic slides. If I have a wonderful slide of Mt. Hood in Oregon and another slide of a mountain in Belgium, placing one slide in front of the other will confuse the picture. I have to move one slide aside to see the other clearly. With homeopathy, we have to try to see what is happening now and what may come next. We must determine what is on top and what is underneath.

Case 1: Man With AIDS

Video Presentation and Case Description

The following discussion was captured as it occurred during a video presentation and case description. Student questions and comments appear within brackets. "HH" indicates a question or comment by Henny Heudens, and "P" indicates "patient."

First Consultation

This man was infected in Africa. First he had syphilis, which was treated with antibiotics. Then he had diphtheria, which also was treated with antibiotics. He had syphilis again, with more antibiotics, and then gonorrhea and more antibiotics. At a certain moment, he got a skin eruption.

He is a chauffeur and must drive hundreds of miles with clients. He sees black spots in his visual field, which makes it dangerous for him to drive the car. He has gotten *Sulphur, Mercurius,* and *Syphilinum,* all of which provided no help. He has skin eruptions in the genital area, where there is an oily sweat, with stinking, which were treated with tea tree oil. Then he got boils with pus and ulcers, with much stinking pus coming out. He has two big complaints in addition to AIDS: He does not sleep well (wakes in the night) and has pain in his legs at night.

I asked him why he went to Africa. "I like to travel, I like hot countries, and I like to make contact with the people. During several months there, I slept with several women." He did not always travel because it was not always possible.

He was a wild boy, daring to do the most extreme things. He was never afraid of anything, and his situation was not easy for his parents to handle. "This is in my family." His mother has osteoporosis, and she cycles hundreds of miles. She must be in her 60s, so she is very likely sycotic.

How does he look? He speaks in quite simple language. How does his mouth look? He likes to kiss. It is a sensual mouth, as if he is always tasting or kissing. It does not belong with the rest of his face. His lips are puckered. He likes to travel, has suppressed genital illnesses, and has a sycotic mother; his symptoms are worse when thinking about them; he has been wild since childhood; he was the one in the class who was sent away from school because of his behavior. The fullness of his lips is a prominent physical feature and indicates the sycotic miasm. [*He looks syphilitic to me.*] Let's see. He is simple and direct in that, if he feels he needs a woman, he takes a woman—like *Sulphur* with a sycotic taint. He had *Sulphur* but did not react because he did not need a psoric remedy. *Sulphur* would not travel from woman to woman. This mouth shows me a man who tastes life, food, and sex. It is nice to learn from the faces of your patients. He is present, feeling his words. He is not philosophizing, just enjoying what he has experienced.

First Prescription

He got a sycotic remedy (*Medorrhinum*) because of his symptoms and because of where he got his disease. He reacted wonderfully to the remedy.

He is not refined; he is as he is. As he says, "When I need something, I take it." He is simple in his language. There is no cruelty, except a history of one fight with his sister as a child. He put the iron in his sister's face, was shocked that he did it, and swore he would never do anything similar again. He also cares for animals. He likes oranges, and he loves dancing.

Second Consultation

After some time, I saw him again, and he continued to improve. Fifteen months later, his eyes were 50 percent better, but he could not sleep at night. He would think about things and brood. He had to get out of bed three or four times every night to urinate and felt tired from lack of sleep. He had to get up early for his job, and waking at night took his energy away. He could not participate in sports anymore. He used to do a lot of sports but hadn't been able to do them for the previous six months.

His nails were breaking, peeling, crumbling, and falling off. Two times in recent weeks he'd had a lot of blood in his stool. He had small ulcers around his anus, from which there was a brown discharge. His penis and testicles had no pus anymore, but there were red spots on the glans; he worried about the spots because he saw that they were becoming holes and growing deeper into his skin. He said, "If this continues, I won't have a penis anymore." He also described pain in the bones of his leg before making stool. He felt better after making stool. He had headaches, as if his head were splitting. On his tongue he had the same spots, like ulcers—holes eating away, aphthae going deep into the tissue.

What do we hear now? [*The syphilitic miasm.*] Did the sycotic remedy work? Yes. His eyes are 50 percent better, as are many other complaints. Now he has a totally different set of symptoms. He needs a syphilitic remedy.

For example, how does he look now? He looks old, weak, and emaciated, and my colleagues all felt he would die. He is not animated at all, but sleepy and dull. "I am weak; I have no energy to do any kind of exertion." After six months, his energy has decreased. I am aware that there may be suppression.

HH—How is your skin?

P—I still have red spots on my thighs, and the eczema came back. (His nails are crumbly and rotten, but only on the left hand.)

HH— How is your temperature?
P—It's normal. I'm not hot, not too cold.
HH—How is your stool?
P—My stool is bad. I have to go to toilet in the morning before work, and when I don't do this I am constipated.

Second Prescription

The remedy he was given is *Kali bichromicum,* a syphilitic remedy. There is a lot of stringy mucus coming from the anus, aphthae in the mouth, and wandering pain in the bones. He has cramps in his calves at night in bed from time to time, and he does not know why. "I never had this before." After the remedy, he started doing exercise again.

Third Consultation

The next time I saw him and asked him how he was eating, he said he was craving chocolate. What is happening with him now? I also asked about alcohol consumption because he seemed very sleepy. He answered my questions slowly, as if he were drunk. He'd been weak like this for some weeks, sleepy and unable to do things. He also has had a lot of thirst. He was almost unable to answer my questions. All of my colleagues felt he was getting worse and worse because he was so weak. The syphilis was much better, only to be replaced with psora—weakness, tiredness, and sleepiness. We have to find the psoric homeopathic remedy that is sleepy, with dry mouth, forgets where he is, and drinks a lot. He had told us that the previous evening he was at a party and a concert and that when he left, he could not find his car. A chauffeur who could not find his car! He walked in the streets and in the woods until he stumbled and fell down. He was so weak, he just slept in the woods. His girlfriend phoned his friends when he did not come home. His friends said he went home early, so they all looked for him. They found him sleeping in the woods, unable to move. In the interview, his eyes were almost closed. He felt as if it were almost impossible to open his eyes, had difficulty thinking, felt cold, had a dry mouth, was unsure of where he was, and was sleepy.

Third Prescription

He gets his psoric remedy, *Nux moschata* 200C. I saw him again a few months later. He was still a bit sleepy but much more lively. He does not get another remedy now. We wait because the remedy is still working. His speaking is livelier, and he is producing symptoms—reacting. [*What about his AIDS?*] His doctor performs tests from time to time, which show amelioration. I saw him again three years after his first consultation (and at times in between). He said he was working all night, so he is tired. He has good color and good reactions. He asked for a remedy for his leg because he needs to drive a long distance. Everything else is fine. All he needs help with is his leg. He is laughing, joking, and minimizing my questions. No remedy here.

A colleague of mine once sent me a holiday wish titled "Patience," whose text was something like, "When you sow a seed in the earth, it will take time before you see the plant. If you see the plant, it will take time before it becomes a tree. When it is a tree, it takes time before there is fruit. When you see the fruit, it takes time before it is ripe. All we need in life is patience." This is how it has to be with homeopathy.

This man is a victim of his disease, and he was declining toward death. During homeopathic treatment, we can see a change in our patients and be unsure whether the change is a good reaction to our remedy. This patient returned after his remedy looking old, weak, and emaciated, as if he would die. He was not animated at all, but sleepy and dull, without enough energy to do anything. If we do not understand the miasmatic response of our patient, we could be concerned by this change in his energy and think that he is less well or that the remedy either did not act or acted badly. When you know how the miasms can appear, you will see that his response is a dramatic change for the better. His vital force is providing symptoms that point to the correct next remedy, and by recognizing the miasms as they surface for treatment, we can follow our patients on their path toward cure.

Remember that our goal is to quiet each miasm, allowing the patient to reach a latent psoric state.

Fourth Consultation

After three years since beginning his treatment, his energy is no problem. He does not run 30 miles anymore as before, but he can do everything else. He does some gymnastics and feels fine. He came this time because his girlfriend left him. He said, "I came to ask you whether you know another one for me. In fact, this is my only problem." He is open, with a dry sense of humor. His girlfriend wanted to see the sexual movies they used to watch, and when he wasn't interested any more, she left him because he was "boring." Now we hear more about the sycotic miasm that was so strong in him before. He gained 25 pounds and feels fine; the only thing he is missing is a woman. He talks about his job and his clients. In fact, he is fine.

Fourth Prescription

The last time I saw him his blood tests were good. He was still alone. He showed some excitement and some desire for alcohol, sweets, and sour things. He slept on his abdomen again and again developed a sycotic picture. *Medorrhinum* was repeated.

Last December he wanted to come back during the seminar, but he was doing so well that there was no need for him to come back. He is fine until now with his *Medorrhinum.* The psoric miasm definitely will emerge again, maybe causing him to have to scratch day and night. We'll have to wait and see what happens before his cure. This is the case after four-and-a-half years. Every time the picture changed, he got the remedy according to his miasmatic state and then according to his symptoms, which brought him into better health. The only thing I am concerned about is the possibility that once he feels really fine and his situation is static, if he has no girlfriend, he might again travel to Africa where there is the possibility to become infected again. I hope he finds a healthy girlfriend so he does not get a new infection. We will warn him that if he again gets an infection, he will need to see his homeopath to get a remedy according to his symptoms and not suppress them with antibiotics because this suppression will cause a relapse in him.

[*Do you think he'll go to Africa again because his sycosis is active?*] He got the infection because of his sexual desire, and at that time he did not know about homeopathy. As long as there is a remaining state of HIV in his blood, he'll be careful. When nothing is found in the blood, he might feel free to do more things, and we have to warn him. With regard to long-term case management, one of my patients with multiple sclerosis felt much better after treatment and was able to walk again. She decided to make the journey of her dreams to an exotic country. Her husband had retired; they had three months of holidays coming up, so she took vaccinations and during the holidays became weaker. She came back in a wheelchair. I warn patients not to waste their energy. They phone and say, "I'd like to ask you a question. We booked holidays, and yesterday I got vaccinations. You agree, right?" They ask me after they do it because they have been feeling so well. When patients with chronic diseases get to the point where they are well, we have to warn them to be careful. Sometimes they will forget how ill they were and how ill they can be again.

We could study this AIDS case for a whole day. I only wanted to show you how miasms change in people. If you are aware of this, you will recognize significance in the changes as they occur. Miasms do not change three times a day but slowly and surely toward better health.

CHAPTER 7

One Diagnosis, Three Disease States

I would like to show you three more cases, all with the same physical disease, multiple sclerosis (MS). We will not go deeply into any of the cases, but I want you to see how each state is individualized by the vital force, even though the diagnosis is the same for each patient. If we were treating in an allopathic way, each would receive the same treatment. Instead we will look at them homeopathically, keeping in mind what we have learned about the influence of miasms and miasmatic prescribing and case management. I will say a little bit about each case as we go along, and you can watch the patients on video.

Case 1: First Woman With MS

Video Presentation and Case Description

The first girl you will see is in her 20s. Her first MS symptoms started before she was 13 years of age; she had difficulty walking and double vision. She had a lot of allopathic treatments, but the illness went on.

What kind of disease is MS? [*Syphilitic, because it is destructive. The nerves are destroyed, and it kills you slowly, sometimes when you are quite young.*] Does this mean that we have to treat MS with syphilitic remedies? [*It depends on how it presents with the patient.*] Right. We don't automatically treat it with a syphilitic remedy because it is a syphilitic disease. That would be allopathy. We have to take the case to see how it has developed. We might see mostly psora or sycosis.

This is a case of a girl who started to get ill very young. What does this mean? [*That she's very weak.*] We are taking this case in front of a group of homeopaths. How is the girl? [*Attractive, lively.*] Yes; how lively? Very. [*She's very attractive.*] How is her makeup? [*Dramatic.*] She moves a lot.

Here are some of the most interesting aspects and her symptoms from her consultation. She makes her own clothing. When she was not quite a teenager, she started to work in a home for old people on Saturdays and Sundays. They liked her very much. She was lively and quick, and this was her life. Then she had a shock.

Be objective. Your reactions are not the patient's reactions.

Many MS patients go through a grief or a shock, then the MS comes. She did not want to talk about it, but finally revealed that her brother had sexually abused her when she was 12 years old. When I asked whether the abuse happened before or after the symptoms were there, she said before. When I asked how she reacted emotionally to this event, she said, "I enjoyed it." I was astonished. She said, "In fact, it was sexually the best period in my life." How is your sexual life now? "Good, but my husband hasn't as much energy as I have." She is quite sensual.

What does she like to do? She designs and makes her own clothes and likes to draw clothes. I asked whether there was anything else. She answered, "Oh yes; I like to dance."

She goes to dances; Look at the video and note how she moves. She also said that she likes to shop. "It is marvelous to be in the shops, to be around the clothes and all the other things a woman likes to have." I asked how she gets to the shops? "I park my car in the handicapped part of the street and walk through the stores. I don't buy anything, but when I see something nice I go home and make it." I asked whether there was anything else she loved to do. "Nothing else special. These are the things I like."

I asked whether she had any fears. She replied, "Oh yes, definitely. I cannot go upstairs to the bathroom when my husband is not at home." What would be the expected answer from someone in her state? "I cannot go upstairs because it is difficult due to my legs." She *fears* going upstairs. I asked her about this fear. "Every time I go upstairs, I'm afraid someone is behind me." In response to my asking about how she sleeps, she said, "on my stomach." She likes to eat oranges.

MS Case 1—Analysis

This patient is clearly in a strongly sycotic state. She needs *Medorrhinum.* This remedy is purely sycotic and covers all of these symptoms; MS is destroying her. We prescribe for the person, not the disease. [*But this is not the person only; this is a syphilitic disease.*] Wonderful! We are thinking in the correct way! But don't be fooled by the disease. If we focus on the fact that the disease is syphilitic, without considering that the person is in her own unique state within this syphilitic disease, we will not be able to help her.

What kind of physical disease do we see? [*Syphilitic.*] Yes. What kind of state do we see? [*Sycotic.*] [*A Medorrhinum state.*] Yes. If we give her a syphilitic remedy because her disease is syphilitic will she be helped? Definitely NOT! If she did not have MS but came instead with stomach ulcers, with the same sleep position, liking to dance, desiring oranges, liking to shop, showing her body off, would this make a difference in the remedy? No.

You have watched only a few minutes of the video to see how she expresses herself, her energy, her sensuality. I have given you her condensed case and characteristic symptoms, which are also keynotes of *Medorrhinum.* This patient has MS, and if she came with these same characteristic symptoms without MS, she would still need her *Medorrhinum.*

When we speak homeopathically about disease, we have to be clear in our understanding. When Hahnemann speaks about what we see in disease, is he talking about the diagnosis as in allopathy? Is this her disease? Why does she have MS? MS is the result of her disease. How severe is her handicap? [*Very severe for being so young.*] Watch her. She has difficulty balancing; she is trying hard to get her energy together, first to stand, and then making the first steps. It took all her energy, but she was smiling. How was she dressed? [*Very tight clothes.*] You could really see the muscles.

If *you* had MS, would you dress yourself in clothing that draws attention to the location of the handicap? Think again about what is typical behavior within the disease of MS. Is it typical to draw attention to your handicap? That is what she is doing. Her black leather trousers draw attention to her body. What is normal when you have a problem? [*To hide the worst.*] What else is strange about her way of walking and moving? Can you imagine her dancing? What is she doing? Again, attracting attention. These are the things she likes to do the most—shopping, dancing, and making her own attractive clothes. When a healthy athletic woman likes these things, it is normal. For this patient, it is a symptom. This is SRP behavior within the disease state, so for her, dancing is a symptom.

Choosing a Symptom

What are the symptoms of MS? [*Weakness, trembling, urinary incontinence, imbalance.*] There is nothing in these symptoms that will help us find a remedy for the patient. When is a symptom a symptom? What makes a symptom a symptom?

[*When the reaction is different from what you would expect in the circumstance.*] Yes. If I were to undress myself here, is that normal? No. If we are at a nightclub and somebody on the stage takes off his or her clothing, is this unusual? It can be, but is there a difference between a nightclub dancer showing herself by undressing and an MS patient showing herself by dancing and wearing tight clothing? For an MS patient, to go dancing is definitely a strong symptom. A nightclub dancer's undressing *may* be a symptom, though not definitely.

When I am teaching you and telling you to be aware, is this a symptom? [*No.*] If I go out to the street and tell the policeman how to do his job because what he is doing is wrong, is that a symptom? Yes, because it is SRP. If a two-year-old child starts to dance as soon as music starts, is that a symptom? No, it is normal. Dancing, shopping, instructing others, taking our clothes off—none are particularly important unless they are SRP for the situation. It is not the symptoms of the MS that are important to us, even though the disease is destructive. When we see what is peculiar for the patient who is suffering in the disease, now we are seeing as homeopaths.

MS Case 1—Followups

We prescribed *Medorrhinum.* Let's see how the case develops. What do you expect from this woman? How will she react to the *Medorrhinum*? [*She'll look more subdued.*] Let's watch her on video. She is a little more nervous about appearing in public. She complains that her legs are not better at all, but she walked up the stairs with no fear anymore in the night. She had forgotten about her fear of going upstairs. She said, "I am growing old. I have started to read books. I never read in my life, and now I am reading books. I want to study something." She is more in the reality of her handicap. She is growing up. How is she dressed? [*More conservatively.*] Yes, in a feminine way. Do you still see or feel or think about a strong sexuality? No, she is still well dressed but not as before. What do you do now? *WAIT* until a new picture comes. It came, and we treated it. Finally, we got her to a syphilitic state for which we gave her a syphilitic remedy. Then her legs were much better. Her mother had MS, her aunt had MS, and her grandmother died of MS; therefore, we see she had a syphilitic background.

What is her miasm? In this case, the three miasms show themselves one by one. She was sycotic in her first state. Then she came in a psoric state.

When she came in a syphilitic state, we treated that state. As homeopaths, we treat what is there until the next miasm comes. This can take years of treatment, which I see in almost all neurological diseases. The treatment takes a long time, but they will come to be in a much better state.

I want to remind you again of Kent's work. He is one of my favorite teachers. Remember that we were discussing Kent's experience with treating hay fever. What is it? Sometimes we give *Allium cepa* to a hay fever patient, but does it cure? Kent says curing a hay fever patient can take four years of treatment. Seventy to 80 years ago it took four years to cure! How has health or disease developed since then? [*Disease is stronger, and people are weaker.*] If we can cure our hay fever patients in less than four years, we are better than Kent. It is unrealistic to think that we can cure these difficult and complicated diseases with one remedy quickly. Fourteen years of MS is impossible to cure in a short time. However, during the period of treatment, the patient must be getting better.

What does Hahnemann say about the quality of homeopathic treatment? [*It should be rapid, permanent, and gentle.*] I agree. If we can stop the disease, we do marvelous work. If we can cure the disease, wonderful. But we cannot do magic. Many homeopaths do not think realistically. Some believe in fairy tales. They want to be magicians and also to be treated by magicians. This is not reality. We have to really understand the disease. This woman's disease is in the tissue. Where there is structural change, it takes much more time to help. This patient is almost fine now. She is walking and dancing. She has studied a lot of things and is now working in a health profession. She is really in balance but is not yet totally cured.

Case 2: Second Woman With MS

Video Presentation and Case Description

Here is another case of MS. Again, what kind of disease is it? Neurological—in the syphilitic miasm. Many of my MS cases are women, which is strange; I have seen few men with this disease. This patient is a 38-year-old woman who has had MS for 20 years. Her situation was considered almost hopeless because of the extensive tissue damage that had occurred over so long a time. A colleague brought her to me because he had not been able to find her remedy.

How does she look? [*Hippocratic face, long chin, sunken teeth.*] She says she has come to me too late. "There is no hope for me to be cured. The doctor advised me to see you. Fifteen years ago you might have been able to do something for me, but now I am a hopeless case, and it is I who made myself ill."

I asked her why? "I'm a thinker." Her husband is with her. He says, "If you could get all the thoughts out of her mind, she would be cured." I asked her what she thinks about. The husband says she thinks about everything. "For example, in the village where we live, people go from house to house to collect money for MS patients to build a clinic for them. But they did not knock on our door, and she got angry. She said 'Why don't they knock at my door? I can give money for this.'"

How is this reaction? This is striking to me, unusual, because it is logical for the fundraisers to not ask her for money for MS because she is afflicted with it. The husband says she gets very angry. He says, "I can see that something is going on, and she does not express it. Then she feels bad, and her MS is bad." He says that she keeps things in. What miasm? Syphilis. He tells us about the miasm without knowing it.

The husband is a very expressive man. He says, "Don't give my wife a remedy for her MS. Give her a remedy not to think so much, and she will be cured." When a husband says this about his wife—the patient— it is very strong. It shows that he sees deeply into the nature of her illness and that she expresses her nature clearly. He is a good man, he takes good care of her, and he does not mind doing it. Can you imagine being in a wheelchair and having to ask your husband for everything?

This is what the woman is saying; this is her reality: She has to ask for help. Her reaction is anger, her way of reacting. She could be grateful or happy she is home with her children. Her expression tells about her state. She is angry but unable to express it immediately. She loses stool and urine. When she is planning to go somewhere, she cannot drink or eat one day before because she cannot contain it when she goes out. Is this logical or not? [*Yes.*]

Let's look at her relationship with her husband. He always responds to her and faces her, but she dismisses him with her suffering. She is afraid that he will leave her. He is loving toward her, and he tries to get her to behave nicely.

The worst moments of her disease are nights. She starts to think how her four children are suffering because their mother has MS. She thinks about how she hates MS. This is strong. A strange thing is that her parents don't know that she has a wheelchair. They live 10 miles away and visit her at least every week; every week when they come, she sits on the couch; the wheelchair is hidden.

She will not talk about her MS or her wheelchair. What is this? [*Hiding.*] This belongs to the syphilitic state.

She is a simple woman. She had worked doing cleaning in hotels. She had done this job until she could no longer stand. Nobody knew she had MS, even though her husband had to pick her up at her workplace. She had almost fallen down and could not come back to work on the weekend. She never told her colleagues about the MS. What is this? Again, the hiding. Why did she not tell? She says, "Because if they knew about my disease and something happened at work, for example, if a little accident occurred where something fell on the floor, they would say, 'It's the lady with MS who did it.' They would blame me." I feel she is suspicious. This is the same feeling she had when people were knocking on other's doors for money and she wondered why she wasn't asked for money. Suspicious.

She said, "Of course, friends of my children don't come to the house because they are afraid of people with MS." What would we do if we had MS? Read, study, do things with our minds. What is she doing? Sitting still and thinking about her disease.

What about watching television? "Sometimes I like it, but I cannot do it all day." And what does she like to watch? "Oh, all those programs about diseases and problems with people."

I asked her whether she reads. She said, "I'm not a reader. I cannot get things in my mind." She is a sensitive woman, but she cannot absorb words in reading. What is that? [*Dullness.*] One of the strong symptoms of the syphilitic miasm is dullness. (This was much better after her remedy. She started to read again.)

She does not drink the whole evening before going to sleep because she would have to wake up her husband to help her go to the toilet. She said that if she did this all the time, her husband would leave her. Watch the husband. He comforts her in a very strong way. She has a nice and wonderful husband, but she does not trust him. This is SRP. Do we have confirmation about the miasmatic state? [*Syphilis*]. And we have to give her a remedy that belongs to the syphilitic state of her mind. Do we have an idea about her remedy?

Why did she develop MS? She fell in love with a boy, and he died in a car accident. "My parents didn't like him. He had to be buried four days after the accident, and I asked my father if I could go to the funeral. My father forbade me to go to the funeral of a stranger. I could not tell my father that I loved this boy." She then told me, "Even my husband does not know that up until now I visited his grave almost every day." How is she hiding and in what way? Her husband says, "But why did you not tell me? I would have taken you to the graveyard." She said she called a taxi on the days he wasn't home, and there at the graveyard she could cry. Do we see why she got MS?

MS Case 2—Analysis

What are her characteristics now? She does not want to be consoled or helped, even when her husband tries. It is strange that this husband has this life. They are at two extremes. The more extreme one is, the more extreme the other.

Remedies? [*I think of remedies such as Natrum muriaticum, Ignatia, Causticum.*] The problem with *Natrum muriaticum* is that it is not a strongly syphilitic remedy. It is more psoric.

Ah-ha! We have syphilitic disease, silent grief, quick anger, dullness of the mind, and guilt. She thinks, "I did this. I am guilty for my disease, and I am guilty that I cannot care for my children."

Is this *Natrum muriaticum*? *Natrum* blames others, not themselves. What is the remedy? A syphilitic remedy that feels guilty for the disease, feels that the disease is her fault, blames herself? The remedy is *Staphysagria.*

MS Case 2—Followups

Two months later, she came back. She is in the wheelchair as before, and she says, "Henny, you cannot believe how I am counting the days to come to you. I don't dare to tell you!" She says that she has written down something that she will give to me to read. She has written a report that she can keep her urine and stool every day. She says, "If you could have done only this for me, I would not have believed it was possible. Now I can go where I want to go. We went out for dinner and enjoyed it." What remedy does she get now? [*Nothing.*]

The case goes on, and some months later she reports to me that she feels more useful in the house because she can peel potatoes and cook. This is progress. She then gets power in her hands to iron the curtains. She cannot do it all at once, but she can do it. This is progress. About six months later, she tells me, "Henny, I wanted to give you a present, but I did not dare." I asked her what it was, and why she did not dare. "I can stand, and I want to show you, but I don't dare." Some time later, she starts to walk.

Even an MS patient of 20 years is improving because she took the remedy belonging to her state and her miasm. It is so helpful to us when we have a framework of understanding. It is nice to see how you can think in cases to find the remedy that helps the patient. She is doing fine now. She is not always walking, but she can stand, goes to the toilet alone, and does a lot of housework. She finally told her parents that she had a wheelchair, and she wanted to show it to them. She said, "Don't be afraid of women in wheelchairs because I am saving money to buy a motorized wheelchair. Then I can go out; my husband can bicycle, I can be in my wheelchair, and I will be happy." Her father said, "I will give you the money for the wheelchair." She is not cured, but she is much better than before. She is useful in her life. She has had several repeats of *Staphysagria* and no other remedy.

Her neurologist told her to go on with her treatment because she was improving. This case is still going on. It is a syphilitic case. Did you know *Staphysagria* is syphilitic? She may remain in a *Staphysagria* state for some time. I know psora will come out, but I cannot see anything else coming yet. All I see is improvement.

Remedy Differentials

Other remedies have been suggested. Let's look at them. What do you see mostly in a *Natrum muriaticum* case? They are very fixed. *Aurum* has silent grief, neurological disturbances, and depression, but she was expressing the fact that she was the cause of her problems. You don't feel that in *Aurum* so much. It is a sign of a *Staphysagria* state to blame oneself.

[*Please differentiate with Causticum.*] They have paralysis and urinary incontinence, but *Causticum* feels more that her family suffers and that she can't do anything for them. "I suffer because I have done something wrong" is *Staphysagria*. Silent grief.

What's the difference between *Aurum* and *Staphysagria*? *Aurum* can be very angry, know they are worth something, and be able to do things; if they take on too much responsibility for the energy they have, they start to have problems. They have high goals and ambition. If she was in an *Aurum* state, I am sure she would read or study. They are very curious. They are industrious, but she sat still. She did not do anything all day. Both have that silence because they are syphilitic.

The difference is that Aurum gets ill because of too much responsibility, and Staphysagria gets ill because of not being able to express feelings.

We see her history, and now we can understand. She did not express her feelings about her boyfriend to her father, and she could not tell her father she was paralyzed. After the remedy, she stopped going to the graveyard; she did not feel the need to go anymore. "I haven't forgotten my friend in my heart," she says. She told her husband that she loved him but that the old boyfriend had been an important part of her life. The case developed well afterward. At this time, the case is only two years old. I need more years, but I see her progressing. I know psora will show itself. How will the itch be if it comes? A big, burning itch may come for at least a year.

She is improving wonderfully. Before she started to walk again, she complained of pain in her legs. She could not stand the pain and asked for something to help. What can you do? Nothing, *definitely nothing*—because sensation is coming back, and this is a sign of her recovery. I never tell a patient that it is wonderful that they suffer, but I told her it might be the life coming back in her legs. After the pain came back, she started to get strength in her legs. I've seen this often with patients who have problems in blood circulation of the veins. Before the situation improves, they go through a period of pain, as if the veins are opening themselves and the structure is changing. If you give them another remedy to cut down the pain, their improvement is finished.

Case 3: Third Woman With MS

Video Presentation and Case Description

This woman is 45 years old, but she looks much older. Her MS started four years ago. We are in the middle of the consultation because in the beginning I did not have the video switched on. Her work was in the medical field, and everything had to be perfect. As a medical professional, she recognizes what happens in MS patients. She says that she has MS and starts to cry very hard because she knows what the end of her disease can be and that no one in her medical profession can help her. So I try to find out how she is.

She is a perfectionist. I try to find out whether there is trouble in the family and where it is. She does a lot, even with the MS. She has her arm hooked in her husband's and walks with difficulty. How did she come to this disease? Why? How is she now, and how was her youth?

Her health was always very good. She was a happy child who lived with her parents, and she was very close to her grandparents. She had the feeling as a child of four that everybody was there to help her—especially her parents and grandparents. She loved her grandfather very much; she would sit on his lap, and he would hold her in his arms, caring for her. She loved getting his support and attention. Grandfather and grandmother moved away to where an uncle of our patient was living. The uncle had children. At a certain time our patient visited her grandparents, went in the house, and saw another child on the lap of her grandfather. She was on holiday and very young (four years old). She developed a fever and became ill the next day. In three days, she lost all her hair. What you see now is not her hair, but a wig. She is bald. It never grew again. She has no eyelashes and no eyebrows. This is her history.

From that day on, she did not dare to go to her grandfather anymore because maybe he would love another child more than her. She remained at her house on a farm and was given some responsibility to feed and care for the pigs. She tells about being very precise. "When a pig would have babies, I was sent to the stable (at 12 years of age) to help. They could rely on me because I was so precise." She has some colds, some coughing, and sometimes the flu, but nothing excessive. She did not consult a homeopath for those problems. Do we have the reason for her MS?

I am sure something else has happened in her life, because she developed MS in her 40s. This is a little late for developing MS. We know something else must have happened in her life. When I asked her about this, she started to cry. She said, "My mother died of cancer, and I cared for her all the time she was ill. I was in her home, and I cared for her until she died. She died in my arms, and I was very happy that I was with her." When I asked her how long ago that was, she said about 10 years ago. The MS started four years ago. Is this the reason for her MS? No; her mother died, but our patient had a good relationship with her; this is not a reason for MS. What else happened? Her marriage is good; her husband is taking care of her and phoning me. Their three children are okay; all are adults and have good jobs. She has a nice house, a nice garden, and a dog. She has every reason to be happy. No problems.

We cannot stop until we understand what happened to our patients and understand their inner state.

I asked her whether something happened four or five years ago. She looked at her husband and started to cry again. She said, "Yes; my father died five years ago." Then her crying was really strong, and I asked her what happened. Her father had remarried, and his second wife did not like our patient. The father got cancer. Our patient phoned her father when she heard about it from her sister. She wanted to visit him. The second wife told her she did not have to care for her father. She said, "I will care for your father. You may visit him for one day, but don't remain here. You must go back because I don't like you." She told our patient this, but not exactly in those words.

Our patient went to see her father that day and saw that he was well cared for. When she went in, the second wife was sitting at the side of his bed with her arm around him, and at that moment our patient was shocked to realize that her father really loved his second wife and wasn't paying much attention to her [our patient]. Exactly the same thing happened that happened with her grandfather when she was four years old, but the difference is she cannot lose her hair anymore; she is already bald. Her body is killing her nerves instead of killing her hair. Could this be a reason to develop MS? I was satisfied. I did not have to know more to find the remedy except a few characteristic symptoms and remarkable things about her life. I knew her inner state.

MS Case 3—Analysis

As we said earlier, there is a logical reason for most illnesses, because the vital force is a logical governing force. Our ability to follow this logic can assist us in understanding the process of disease in our patients. We know that this patient reacted on seeing her grandfather caring for another person—feeling that, because he cared for another, he did not love her anymore, and reacting with physical illness. This happened again 5 years ago when she saw her father's love for his second wife. She felt that he loved her less because he loved his wife. This is the weakness in her. Her susceptibility is the feeling of being rejected, not being good enough, not being loved; somebody is preferred in her place. We need a remedy that has this possibility, this susceptibility.

What else do we need in the remedy? [*The baldness.*] Is it normal to lose all your hair from an emotional situation? [*How often have you seen a case like that?*] Not very often, perhaps three or four cases.

What miasm is this? [*Psora.*] She is weak emotionally, and immediately the emotions go very deep inside. How else is she? [*Fastidious.*] We see that in how she expresses herself—crying a lot, affectionate. [*Caring for others.*] She is very precise. Is she really jealous? Jealous people who are sycotic scream, shout, and make a big scene. What did she do? She stepped backward and did not show herself anymore. She is cold and always has cold feet.

What psoric remedy is very cold, bald, and fastidious; withdraws herself; feels forsaken and cries easily? [*Baryta carbonica has all these symptoms.*] [*Silica is another possibility.*] This patient was brand-new to homeopathy. She has never taken a homeopathic remedy. *Baryta carbonica* was the best choice for her. Better than *Silica,* which is very close. [*She also looked a lot older.*] It is nice to see now what the remedy did for her.

MS Case 3—Followups

Watch the video. The first thing we notice is her walking. Now she is more angry than she is sad or depressed as before. Her energy is better than before—she does not get tired as fast. How else is she? She had a headache. What's the difference between the first consultation and this one? [*She is now happy and relaxed.*] She looks younger. How is her behavior? She seems to be happy, not complaining. She is saying that she got a headache and hiccups after the remedy. She gives a detailed report about what was going on. *Arsenicum, Baryta carbonica,* and *Silica* can all give this kind of detailed report. The language she uses now is more childish than before. She looks younger, more like *Baryta carbonica* now.

When somebody did something to her before that she did not like, she kept it in; now she reacts. She is less tolerant of others. She describes her nights as very good. She gets up very early to prepare everything in the home. When she feels tired, it is usually in the middle of the day—psora! I asked her how she felt emotionally and what influences her emotions. She says she is more like she was before the MS. I asked about her MS symptoms later on.

How did she react to the remedy? Psychologically, she's much better. Physically, she has pain in the eyes only now and then. This was worse before. She can take off her glasses sometimes. In the beginning of the disease, she had poor peripheral vision; now it is better. She's driving her car again. She did not have enough strength in her feet before. Now that her vision and strength are better, she can focus again. How is her balance? She walks better and faster now. She can walk alone, although her lower legs feel stiff. She adds, "My eyebrows and eyelashes are coming back since last time."

Did the remedy work? [*Yes.*] She has needed one repeat of the remedy, and I will see her again. She phoned last week and said she was improving. She speaks enthusiastically. The first time she was hanging on her husband, lifting her legs just high enough to walk. Now she is quick in moving her feet. This is a psoric remedy helping her over her disease. I hear that her hair is growing now.

The wonderful thing is that you can entertain theories, but you can only know whether your reasoning was correct when you see the patient again. You must see whether your thinking was right.

[*Baryta carbonica was in the rubric,* DELUSION; deserted, *which is what she felt with the father and grandfather.*] It shows how weak her energy was. Can you imagine a child who sees someone she loves caring for another and getting so ill that she loses all her hair? This shows how low her energy was, and now it is stronger. In what way is she stronger?

[*She is stronger because she is able to express a level of anger.*] The term she used was "upsetting." She reacts now to upset or anger. She is expressing.

She was stuck at four years of age, and now she gets over it at the age of 46 years. She is not cured yet, but I've been treating her for one year. The improvement is very good so far.

Remedy Differentials

In such a case we can struggle between remedies—*Silica*? *Baryta carbonica*? I knew she needed a psoric remedy. *Silica* and *Tuberculinum* are with *Baryta carbonica* in the same rubric in *The Complete Millennium*: HEAD; HAIR; *affections of, in general; baldness; young people. Lycopodium* is one of the remedies in the rubric for baldness in patches. However, *Lycopodium* is a trimiasmatic remedy, and *Silica* has a lot of syphilis.

Baryta carbonica is known as one of the largely psoric remedies. Why do we choose *Baryta* for this patient? We have a lot of symptoms for *Silica*. There are fewer for *Lycopodium*. How would *Lycopodium* behave in this situation? *Lycopodium* reacts by showing strength in another way and hiding the weakness and trying to overcome it by doing other things. This is why they are sometimes teachers. We see the weakness of *Lycopodium* a lot in our practice. Summer holidays are from July 1 to September, and on July 3 the teachers start calling on the phone. They have their consultations, and they complain about their anxiety—having only two months until school starts again. Does this patient have this anticipation of *Lycopodium* or *Silica*? No, but anticipation is a big thing in *Lycopodium* and in *Silica*.

How was this patient with her grief? If she needed *Lycopodium*, she would do something to get the grandfather's attention. She would *make* him look at her. If she needed *Silica*, what would she do? She'd be pitiful, looking for comfort or sympathy or support from someone else to lift her up. Do we hear this? Did she have that reaction? Not at all. What did she do? She withdrew. She suffered.

Baryta carbonica looks for support only when she cannot do things alone. She has anxiety about trifles, and the things she can do, she does wonderfully and correctly. *Baryta carbonica* is seldom a true intellectual.

If you have three children all needing these different remedies, and you tell them it is time to go to sleep, get all their toys together, and put them where they belong, what will they do? *Lycopodium* will make the others do it; he'll dictate. *Baryta carbonica* will put away things piece by piece. *Silica* will tell his mother "yes," and then do nothing. He'll let *Baryta carbonica* do it.

Concluding Remarks on MS Cases

So many times in these difficult diseases, the miasmatic knowledge has helped me find the remedy and understand the patient. I am very aware of signs and symptoms of the miasms that can be recognized in patients. Therefore, I wanted to show you these three videos. I could have shown you the same thing with warts, itching, or appendicitis, but now you have you seen this kind of miasmatic assessment for MS, a more difficult diagnosis.

CHAPTER 8
CONCLUSION

All homeopathic remedies have the potential to touch a person's state in a profound way, to stimulate the vital force to return to health. Can we be good homeopaths without miasmatic prescribing? The patient herself can take a homeopathic remedy for a specific set of symptoms, and possibly this is the remedy that will help her deeply. The novice prescriber can sometimes find wonderful remedies for his patients, even though just a beginner. So why bother trying to understand our patients from a miasmatic perspective? As those of us who have been in practice for even a year know, it is not always the first prescription that is the most difficult. Knowing what to do when the patient returns and has not reacted to our remedy or has reacted and is not better or has reacted well but stops improving or is in a different state—this is when homeopathy becomes more complicated.

Remember the goal set forth by our founder, Samuel Hahnemann, as stated in the *Organon, 6th edition.*

> *"The highest ideal of therapy is to restore health rapidly, gently, permanently; to remove and destroy the whole disease in the shortest, surest and least harmful way, according to clearly comprehensible principles."* (Organon of Medicine, *Aph 2)*

With this as our goal, our knowledge of the nature of chronic disease and miasmatic case management can greatly increase the chances of our being successful in practice. It is not learned overnight, any more often than cure occurs overnight. Cure in this way is an art and can take years of fearless attention and focus on the part of the homeopath.

The disease complexes in our patients today are much more complicated and more difficult to treat than they were 100 years ago because of widespread vaccination, medical innovations, and suppressions. Knowing that there are limitations and knowing the complexity of chronic disease today, we cannot expect that one remedy will cure our patient, that he will live well into old age without trouble. This sometimes happens, but the rest of the time curing our patients is hard work.

Getting to the "Basis" of Disease

The basis of disease includes the history of the patient back through childhood and even before birth—in the womb and through the ancestral heritage. These things have already been discussed, but for this discussion, I use the words "basis of disease" to mean the state of the person just before he got his disease. We must treat that state, that disturbance, and all of the miasms in his "rucksack" that have contributed to that state, if we are to fully restore this patient to health. Because his state is made up of everything in the "miasm pot," we must treat these miasms to fully cure the patient.

Suppose a patient has a heart attack with pain in both arms. We prescribe *Latrodectus mactans*. The patient feels a little better but then has another heart attack. This means that we were treating the heart and not the state. To understand and treat the state, we must discover that state of the patient in the days before this event happened. Maybe we will find a *Lycopodium* (tri-miasmatic remedy) patient with a lot of anticipation and nervousness. What has *Latrodectus* done in the best scenario? Perhaps saved his life. But the remedy that is prescribed for his state before the heart attack will strengthen his whole organism so he will be healthier.

If *Lycopodium* acts for a while but fails to continue in effect, we may see things that have changed in him: Now he is much more talkative, he feels strongly jealous, and he cannot lie on his left side. Now we see a totally new picture—a new state—*Lachesis* (predominantly syphilitic miasm). The *Lycopodium* state could have grown on the *Lachesis* state that was underneath, and once Lycopodium completes its effect, the new state, *Lachesis*, comes forward. After he receives *Lachesis*, the danger of him having another heart attack has lessened greatly. Now a heart attack is unlikely. He is safer after the *Lachesis* than he was after the *Lycopodium*.

Because we are managing his treatment with miasmatic consideration and we know that his father had a history of gonorrhea or strongly sycotic behavior, we are always watching closely for symptomatic expressions of the miasms that he has inherited from his parents. If he stops reacting to *Lachesis* and his symptom picture shifts to characteristics of *Medorrhinum*, we are not surprised. When we give *Medorrhinum*, we arrive at the real basis of his disease—perhaps the last remedy he will need for his system to become stable—and then return him to the latent psoric state. If we can reach this place in our patients, they'll be fine. Latent psora is the healthiest possible state.

The Progression of Miasms

We know that patients can carry more than one miasm, and we must treat the miasm that is on top—the one showing most strongly. Let's look one last time a little more closely at treating miasms as they profess themselves more strongly at different times.

In our discussion of sycosis, the female patient comes to us with recurring bladder infections, pain in the abdomen, and green leucorrhoea. She tells us she itches a lot, but mostly she does not feel well in the abdomen. She stays up late at night, is very weak in the morning, but is active in the night. She is sycotic. We want to prescribe a sycotic remedy. She is cold, worse wet weather, and stiff, with fixed ideas and a feeling of fragility. *Thuja* will help her.

After the *Thuja*, she will sleep better. She may get tired earlier in the evening and have to go to bed earlier. Some months go by, and at some point she may begin to lie awake thinking about her children, what she will feed them in the morning, what she can do to earn more money, and how she will be able to go to the homeopathic seminar that costs so much. In her sycotic state, she went to seminars and went dancing afterward. Now she worries, feels a little cold, has to cover herself, and starts to perspire on the neck. Her feet get so cold she has to put on socks. Now her psora has come to the surface.

Her sycosis has calmed down, and psora has become more prominent. Is this good? Yes. Maybe she does not like it initially, but we homeopaths are very happy with her progress because she has come back to psora. We can now treat the active psora, and she will become healthier. Always, we prescribe on the current state and follow the case to see how it develops. We treat the miasms as they come up, in whatever order (and there is no set order), until the patient can return to a latent psoric state. If we cannot unravel the miasmatic puzzle, we will never get our patients to this stable state.

Recognizing SRP Symptoms and the Miasm Needing Treatment

When more than one miasm is represented in a patient's symptoms, finding the most SRP expressions or symptoms will often "shoot" to the miasm that is most asking for treatment at the time of the consult. I am the patient now. Let's say I have a fear of mice. Sometimes I kill an insect. Sometimes I like to drink wine. It is so nice to celebrate. I find out that three glasses of wine are more than enough. I get a little tipsy, but still I like that third glass. Whenever I go outside in the cold air, I cough. When I see some nice green leaves coming out on a tree in the spring, I start to cry. Here, I have shown a symptom from each of the miasms, and I have more symptoms from each one. My homeopath must choose the most SRP symptom(s):

- Fear of mice—A lot of people fear mice.
- Killing an insect—Not very unusual.
- Drinking one glass of wine too many with a celebration—This does not make me sycotic.
- Coughing when it is cold—A fairly common problem in winter.
- Crying when I see the green leaves of spring—How many people do this?

Weeping at the beauty of nature. This is SRP. Of course, we are theorizing here—a simple example to make a point.

When a reaction is different from one we would normally see in a certain situation or when it is not necessarily unusual but very definitely out of proportion, it is a symptom.

Remember to consider the culture as well as the situation to decide what is SRP. When a Turkish woman says that she does not go to a pub with her husband, this is not unusual. But if a Belgian wife says this, we would have to ask her why. If an Iranian woman throws herself down on the ground to weep and wail from grief, it is not a symptom; it is cultural. If a British woman does this, it is a symptom. Find out what the patient is doing that is not according to the culture. These are often important symptoms.

The Path to Cure

If there are several miasms in a patient's case, she will rarely need only one remedy. I say rarely, because sometimes one remedy is broad enough to cover several miasms and can act for a long time, and if she leaves our practice before she dies, we may not know if she needs something else in her future. I have a patient who is also a homeopath, and she had a strong history of severe asthma as a child, a strong need for change, and desire for fresh air and excitement. She has had a primarily psoric remedy, followed by a primarily sycotic remedy, then a tiny bit of psoric remedy again and another psoric remedy. She has a family history of tuberculosis, and since I have been treating her during the last seven years, none of her asthmatic symptoms have returned. She questioned me as to why: if my theories of miasmatic prescribing are true, why has she never needed a tubercular remedy? I replied that she is not dead yet.

The patient may come to us in an active psoric state. After the remedy, the sycotic symptoms may come to the top, and then we need to treat what is there until the next miasm comes up. Some cases will have more miasms than others. A few patients may go back and forth between miasms until cure comes. Each time a miasm surfaces in a patient, its symptomatic expression will tend to be more superficial than when the patient first came for treatment.

Treatment can take time. I have the feeling that we homeopaths are not always grounded in reality; we know the power of the correctly prescribed homeopathic remedy, and we want to be magicians who can cure overnight.

> *It is neither the homeopath nor the remedy that cures the patient. Cure is possible only through the power of the vital force. The vital force will take its own time to cure.*

When a remedy is the simillimum, it will start to work as soon as it touches the patient. How soon the patient feels better depends on the patient and her vital force. Do not be distracted by her every minor complaint. Is her energy better, is she sleeping, is she working, is she having some enjoyment? If so, we must leave her alone. The quality of the patient's energy and sleep is very important after the remedy. We also have Hering's rules on which to rely: from the inside out, from top to bottom, old symptoms returning. These rules help us know whether the healing process is going in the right direction.

We have to be cautious in prescribing. If things are still changing a lot, WAIT—let the vital force continue its work.

Hering says that when there is an aggravation, improvement, and then an aggravation again—WAIT. Then we will see a most marvelous cure. In the *Organon,* Hahnemann tells us that if we administer the correct homeopathic remedy, the patient can get an aggravation, then amelioration, and then in **six weeks** we can expect to see that the illness is again fighting with the vital force. Here we must wait—the vital force will win; the cure will be there. I see my patients for followup after two months, because I am afraid that if I see them at six weeks, I will give them a remedy. Hering and Hahnemann both warned about this.

When we see a lot of amelioration but everything is not yet well, we must WAIT until we see a true relapse or until a new picture emerges.

Cure rarely happens in a straight line. A patient became ill in steps; so too, will she get well in steps. Her energy will fluctuate up and down a little on the way to cure. If her energy is going up in a wavy line, good. Do not jump in to prescribe for every complaint and spoil the progress. No one always has energy in a steady line. When the energy of the patient is standing still and not improving anymore or when there has been a true relapse, we can give a remedy again. Do not change the remedy for one new symptom—only if the state has really changed. If the energy is going down in a wavy line, then there is a problem, and we must analyze the case again, as there may be a new remedy or a better remedy. Objective observation. What is happening? What is needed?

We've all heard about obstacles to cure. Sometimes we homeopaths are our own obstacles to cure.

Sometimes the patient is telling us his symptoms, and we are thinking of rubrics and remedies instead of trying to understand the patient. We know what we need to do—listen to the symptoms and base our remedy choice on those that are characteristic. Ask questions until we understand the case. We make simple things complicated by theorizing. We get into "maybe this" and "maybe that" and become lost even though we have an abundance of wonderful symptoms to guide us. If we make a list of what is sure and do not speculate, we will see the remedy clearly.

What Influences Your Miasmatic Prescription?

We need to answer the following questions when deciding which miasm needs to be treated:

- Which miasm is the strongest right now?
- Which miasm was strongest when the patient was born?
- Which miasm(s) run(s) through the family history? We need a complete family history of diseases—parents and grandparents on both sides of the family—to know the family weaknesses.
- What are the most unusual symptoms (not the common symptoms of the disease but those that are strange, rare, and peculiar [SRP])?
- Which miasm do these represent?
- What are the modalities that run throughout the case, and which miasms are indicated in these modalities?

To determine the correct remedy, we must focus our choice of rubrics on the most characteristic SRP symptoms, taking into consideration the miasm that is most prominent in the patient and therefore that most limits the patient's overall well-being at the time of treatment. So simple is miasmatic case management.

Fearless Perseverance

When miasms overlap, it is confusing and difficult to see a clear picture, but don't get discouraged: The ability to see clearly will come with practice. When I finished my (initial) study of homeopathy, I thought I might cure the entire world. After the first year, I was doing quite well, but with each year a little bit less so. At the end of the fourth year, I thought I would quit because it was too difficult. It was as if I had become color blind—unable to discern one remedy from the next, one set of characteristic symptoms from another. Then a patient came back and said how very well he was. I thought, "Perhaps I *can* do this. How hard can it be?" How naïve.

Homeopathy is very complicated. I don't think there is another profession that requires so much of the practitioner. We have to see clearly, listen carefully, smell and sometimes touch, know ourselves, and face our fears about being present with a patient and about being in practice. We must remove our own prejudices, know what is normal behavior in a given situation, make notes, study in our books or on our computers, understand, analyze, and sometimes be a kind of Sherlock Holmes to understand between the lines—all of this from one consultation. This is quite a lot to do and for me, has meant a lifetime of practice. But it is the understanding of the miasms that has contributed most to what success I have been able to accomplish.

So here we are, at the end of the seminar, with a few principles and some examples of how to use the knowledge of the miasms in case analysis and case management as a way to help our patients overcome their basic chronic weaknesses and jump to their best level of health.

We are so fortunate in homeopathy that, instead of relying on medical fashion, we have homeopathic rules that have been practiced successfully for 200 years. By following the teachings of Hahnemann, we can do this wonderful work that he has given us. If we take his lead in understanding the miasms and use this knowledge in our practices, our results will greatly improve. I encourage all homeopaths to love their work and its potential to heal at this deepest level. I wish you much success in your work with the miasms.

APPENDICES

Appendix 1: Comparative Summary of the Chronic Miasms

The following brief summaries are meant to give hints of the general tendencies of each miasm. Remember that, ultimately, every symptom must be understood in context.

1. GENERAL TENDENCIES AND ENERGY OF THE CHRONIC MIASMS

Psora

- The idea of too little
- Deficiency
- Weakness
- Slow reaction
- Slow growth
- Low energy
- Poor assimilation

Syphilis

- The idea of destruction
- Perversion
- Deformation
- Hidden reaction
- Hidden growth
- Mostly normal energy

Sycosis

- The idea of too much
- Excess
- Sudden reaction
- Overreaction
- Rapid growth
- High energy

Tubercular

- The idea of travel
- Change
- High energy in bursts—then worn out
- Elements of psora, syphilis, and sycosis

Cancer

- The idea of perfectionism
- Extreme sensitivity
- Suppression
- Energy a little up and down
- Elements of psora, syphilis, sycosis, and tuberculosis

2. MENTAL AND EMOTIONAL TENDENCIES OF THE CHRONIC MIASMS

Psora

- Many fears/anxieties
- Guilt, shame, embarrassment
- Sensitive feelings
- Inhibited, shy
- Needs and wants support
- Dependent
- Can be too tired for sex
- Prefers light conservative colors—beige, blue, gray

Syphilis

- Dullness of mind and emotion
- Absence of guilt, shame, embarrassment
- Disconnected from feelings
- Silent
- Self-contained
- Isolated
- Secretive
- Closed
- Harbors hatred and revenge

- Capable of perverted sexual behavior
- Likes dark colors—brown, black

Sycosis

- Likes excitement—"kicks"
- Showy—wants attention
- Open, outgoing, friendly
- Impatient
- Hurried
- Bossy
- Shows extremes of feeling
- Independent
- Takes action
- Lots of sexual feelings, sexual activity
- Likes bright colors—red, yellow, orange

Tubercular

- Seeks excitement—new experiences—new places
- Sensitive feelings, particularly in artistic ways—art, music, etc.
- Bossy
- Temper tantrums
- Hopeful (even in disease)
- Fear or dislike of animals
- Loves fresh air and mountains

Cancer

- Very sensitive feelings
- Careful not to hurt feelings of others—suppression of own feelings
- Caring
- Self-sacrificing
- Perfectionistic
- Fastidious—especially about beauty of surroundings
- Very sensitive to beauty and nature, cries in reaction to them
- Loves animals
- Loves to dance

3. CHARACTERISTIC MODALITIES OF THE CHRONIC MIASMS

Psora

- Worse movement
- Better morning and evening
- Worse midday
- Worse cold
- Better warmth

Syphilis

- Worse drafts, wind
- Worse too hot or too cold
- Worse sunset to sunrise
- Better day

Sycosis

- Better movement
- Better twilight and night
- Worse morning and day
- Worse warmth/Better cold

Tubercular

- Worse wet and damp
- Better from movement but tires easily
- Better at night

Cancer

- Energy used up quickly
- Better at the sea

4. PHYSICAL TENDENCIES OF THE CHRONIC MIASMS

Psora

- Skin problems
- Psoriasis
- Itching, burning, dryness, sweating
- Disorders of sensation and function
- Physical sensitivity

- Sour smells
- Seeks rich, high calorie foods

Syphilis

- Bone pains/coldness
- Bleeding and blood diseases
- Deformations, holes in tissue, cracks in skin
- Physical insensitivity
- Stinking smells
- Likes cold food and drinks and smoked (deadened) foods (tubercular)

Sycosis

- Growths
- Warts
- Swelling, inflammations, suppurations, and catarrh
- Genital and urinary problems
- Physical overreaction
- Fishy smells
- Prefers strong-tasting, spicy foods

Tubercular

- Respiratory problems, allergies, tendency to colds, coughs
- Elevated temperature and sweating (especially on chest)
- Paleness/flushes on cheeks
- Narrow chest with prominent chest bone
- Emaciation
- Likes ice cream, cold milk, burnt (barbequed) foods (syphilitic)

Cancer

- Café au lait spots, blue sclera
- Chronic fatigue
- Mononucleosis
- Adult disease in childhood, childhood diseases in adults
- Very destructive diseases
- Family history of diabetes, cancer
- Possibility for AIDS
- Loves chocolate

Appendix 2: Comparative Chart Miasmatic Tendencies and Expressions

1. General Tendencies and Energy within the Chronic Miasms

Psora	Syphilis	Sycosis	Tubercular	Cancer
• Idea of too little • Deficiency • Weakness • Slow reaction • Slow growth • Poor assimilation • Low energy	• Idea of destruction. • Perversion • Deformation • Hidden reaction • Hidden growth • Mostly normal energy	• Idea of too much • Excess • Sudden reaction • Overreaction • Rapid growth • High energy	• Idea of travel • Change • Elements of psora, syphilis, and sycosis • High energy in bursts, then worn out	• Idea of perfectionism • Extreme sensitivity • Suppression • Elements of psora, syphilis, sycosis, and tuberculosis • Energy up and down

2. Characteristic Modalities of the Chronic Miasms

Psora	Syphilis	Sycosis	Tubercular	Cancer
• Worse movement • Better morning and evening • Worse midday • Worse cold • Better warmth	• Worse drafts, wind • Worse too hot or too cold • Worse sunset to sunrise • Better daytime	• Better movement • Better twilight and night • Worse morning and day • Worse warmth • Better cold	• Worse wet and damp • Better from movement but tires easily • Better at night	• Energy used up quickly • Better at the sea

3. MENTAL AND EMOTIONAL TENDENCIES WITHIN THE CHRONIC MIASMS

Psora	Syphilis	Sycosis	Tubercular	Cancer
• Many fears—anxiety • Guilt, shame, embarrassed • Sensitive feelings • Inhibited, shy • Needs and wants support • Dependent • Can be too tired for sex • Prefers light conservative colors—beige, blue, gray	• Dullness • Absence of guilt, shame, chagrin • Discon-nected from feelings • Silent • Self-contained • Isolated • Secretive • Closed • Harbors hatred and revenge • Capable of perverted sexual behavior • Prefers dark colors—brown, black	• Creates excitement • Showy—wants attention • Open, outgoing, friendly • Impatient • Hurried • Bossy • Shows extremes of feeling • Independent • Takes action • Lots of sex-ual feelings and sexual activity • Loves or hates animals and can be abusive • Likes bright colors—red, yellow, orange	• Seeks excite-ment, new experi-ences/places • Sensitive feelings, par-ticularly in artistic ways—art, music • Demanding • Temper tantrums • Hopeful (even in disease) • Fear or dislike of animals • Loves fresh air and mountains	• Very sensitive feelings • Careful not to hurt feelings of others, sup-presses his own feelings • Caring • Self-sacrificing • Perfectionist, fastidious, especially about beauty of surroundings • Very sensitive to beauty and nature, cries in reac-tion to beauty and nature • Loves animals • Loves to dance

4. PHYSICAL TENDENCIES WITHIN THE CHRONIC MIASMS

Psora	Syphilis	Sycosis	Tubercular	Cancer
• Skin problems • Psoriasis • Itching, burning, dryness, sweating • Disorders of sensation and function • Physical sensitivity • Sour smells • Seeks rich, high calorie foods	• Bone pains • Cold pain • Bleeding and blood diseases • Deformations, holes in tissue, cracks in skin • Physical insensitivity • Stinking smells • Prefers cold food/drinks • Smoked food (tuberc.)	• Growths • Warts • Swelling, inflammations, suppurations, and catarrh • Genital and urinary problems • Physical overreaction • Fishy smells • Prefers strong tasting, spicy foods	• Respiratory problems, allergies, tendency to colds, coughs • Elevated temperature and sweating (especially on chest) • Paleness • Flush on cheeks • Narrow chest with prominent chest bone • Emaciation • Desires ice cream, cold milk • Burnt (barbequed) foods (syph)	• Café au lait spots • Blue sclera • Chronic fatigue • Mononucleosis • Adult diseases in childhood • Childhood diseases in adults • Tendency to destructive diseases • Family history of diabetes, or cancer • Desires chocolate

INDEX

A

ABNORMAL DEVELOPMENT 159–160
ABUSE, SEXUAL 17, 64, 216
ACTIVE MIASMS 3–5
ACUTE SITUATIONS 107
ADDICTIONS
  alcohol 65, 76, 85, 97
  drugs 65, 149
  gambling 65, 124–125, 126, 131–132
ADHD (ATTENTION DEFICIT HYPERACTIVE DISORDER) 51–52, xiii
ADULT DISEASES IN CHILDREN 156, 182, 189–190, 198
AGE OF PATIENTS 36, 193
AGGRAVATIONS 37, 41, 236. *See also* individual causes; Modalities
AGGRESSION 54, 58, 73, 164–165
AIDS (ACQUIRED IMMUNE DEFICIENCY SYNDROME) 205–206, 208–214
ALCOHOL 18, 60, 70–71, 111
ALCOHOLISM 65, 76, 85, 97
ALLERGIES 148, 154, 158–169, 219
ALLOPATHIC THINKING IN HOMEOPATHS 105, 107, 169, 175, 185
ALLOPATHIC TREATMENT
  contrasted to homeopathy 139–140, 161
    anxiety 178
    ear infections 67
    MS 215
    tuberculosis 146
  suppressive medication 6, 205–206
    asthma 148
    canker sores 68
    gonorrhea 121
    kidney or intestinal problems 74
    teething problems 26
    thrush 77, 78
ALZHEIMER'S DISEASE 66–67
AMELIORATIONS 37, 236. *See also* individual causes; Modalities
ANEMIA, PERNICIOUS 189, 190
ANGER
  cases with 174, 196–204, 220
  psoric ineffectual 18
  syphilitic extreme 59, 73
ANIMALS
  cruelty to 153
  dogs chosen by miasms 20, 111, 141
  extreme concern for 187–188, 201–203
  fear of 150, 153, 157
  love of 47–48, 110–111, 136–137, 138, 192
ANTIBIOTICS 26, 140, 147, 155, 170, 176
ANTIDEPRESSANTS 16, 58, 70
ANTIDOTING REMEDIES 41–42
ANTIMONIUM TARTARICUM 99–100
ANXIETY 15–16, 19, 20, 28, 201
APGAR SCORES 77, 94, 97, 103–104
APHTHAE 68, 77, 136, 137, 210
APPEARANCE
  cancerous/carcinosin 181–182, 191
  causing mistakes in prescribing 34
  psoric 17–18
  sycotic 115, 118, 137
  syphilitic 62, 70
  tubercular 154
APPENDICITIS 25, 119
ARGENTUM 123
ARGENTUM NITRICUM 114
ARNICA 99–100, 101–103
ARSENICUM 81, 188
ARTISTIC INCLINATIONS 145–146, 149, 152, 153
"AS IF" SENSATIONS 23
ASSIMILATION, POOR 20, 21, 23, 239
ASTHMA 9–10, 22, 47, 98, 119
ASYMMETRY 65, 70
ATHLETES 148–149
ATTENTION DEFICIT-HYPERACTIVE DISORDER (ADHD) 51–52, xii
ATTENTION, DESIRE FOR 122, 217
AURUM METALLICUM 76, 140, 223–224
AUTISM 89, 94, 106–107
AUTOIMMUNE DISEASES 69
AWAKENING MIASMS 4–6

B

BACILLUS CALMETTE-GUERIN (BCG) VACCINE 135, 137, 147
BAD NEWS AS DISEASE TRIGGER 4–6, 216
BARYTA CARBONICA 227–228, 229

BEAUTY, SENSITIVITY TO 187, 188–189
BEAUTY, TUBERCULAR 145, 153, 155
BED-WETTING 29, 39, 45
BEHAVIOR DISORDERS 51–52
BIRTH DEFECTS 74, 79
BLAND DISCHARGES 20, 22
BLOCKED CASES 10, 157–158, 192
BLOOD PRESSURE 24, 69, 122, 178
BLOODY DISCHARGES 65
BLUE SCLERA 153–154, 181, 183, 189–190
BLUENESS 99, 101–103, 153, 156
BOASTING 8, 110, 111
BODY PIERCING 63, 115
BONE COMPLAINTS 23, 65, 66, 70–71, 74, 76
BORAX 77, 100
BOSSINESS 111, 122, 156, 187
BREAK OBJECTS, URGE TO 152–153
BUNGEE JUMPING 113, 152
BURNING 8, 21

C

CAFE AU LAIT SPOTS 183, 189, 190
CALCAREA ARSENICOSA 157
CALCAREA CARBONICA
  considered in cases 27, 40, 49, 185
  miasmatic composition 7–8, 11, 34
  symptoms 14–15, 189
CALCAREA PHOSPHORICA 81, 156, 157
CALCULATIONS, DIFFICULTY DOING 76
CAMPHORA 99
CANCER (DISEASE)
  causes 74, 148, 183, 185, 186
  distinguished from miasm 184–186
  family history of 85, 91, 181–182
  treating 192–195
CANCER (MIASM) 181–204
  distinguished from disease 184–186
  in infants and children 181–184
  mental and emotional symptoms 186–189
  physical symptoms and modalities 189–190
  remedies 190–192
CANNABIS 206–207
CARBO VEGETABILIS 100
CARCINOSIN
  appearance 181–183
  and cancer disease 185, 190, 192
  given in cases 201–204
  symptoms 156, 186, 187, 189, 190
CARS, BUYING 19–20, 62, 111
CASE MANAGEMENT
  application of miasms 10–11, 231, xii
  blocked cases 157–158, 192
  interviewing 54, 125
  prescribing 234, 237
CAUSTICUM 114, 125, 127, 128, 223
CHANGEABILITY 114, 149, 156
CHEERFULNESS 145
CHEESE, SMELL OF OLD 118, 119
CHEMOTHERAPY 192–193
CHESTS, NARROW 153, 154, 155
CHILDISHNESS 17, 33, 96, 99
CHILDREN
  with cancer miasm 181–184
  loyalty to parents 165
  psoric 15, 25–28
  sycotic 111, 122–123
  syphilitic 72–74
  treat to protect next generation 139
  tubercular 155–156
  urge to kill ones own 57–58, 64
CHILDREN'S DISEASES 183–184, 189, 203
CHINA 99
CHOCOLATE, LOVE OF 189, 192, 211
CHRONIC DISEASE 1–2, 213–214
CHRONIC FATIGUE 190
CITIES, LOVE OF 112, 126
CLAIRVOYANCE 196, 201
CLEAR DISCHARGES 20, 22
CLINGING 13, 25, 44, 136
CLOSED NATURE 55, 170–171
CLOTHING CHOICES 17–18, 62, 115, 188–189
COFFEE 42
COLD AGGRAVATES 25, 28, 242
COLD FOODS AND DRINKS, DESIRE FOR 66, 153, 154, 156
COLDNESS
  psora 17, 21–22, 28, 34
  syphilis 78–79, 243, 246
  tuberculosis 153, 156
COLDS 25, 26–27, 126, 154
COLIC IN INFANTS 123, 135
COMPLAINTS, MINOR 235–236
COMPULSIVE BEHAVIOR 56, 98, 99, 117–118
CONFIDENCE, LACK OF 19
CONNECTION, LACK OF 55–56, 62, 95, 98–99, 199
CONSCIENTIOUSNESS ABOUT TRIFLES 18
CONSOLATION 17, 62, 72, 76
CONSTIPATION 8, 23, 25, 26, 90
CONTAMINATION, FEAR OF 76

CONTRADICTORY SYMPTOMS 150, 153
CONVULSIONS 158–169
CORROSION 65, 67
COUGHING 29–39, 145, 154, 157, 164–169
CRACKS 65, 69, 72
CROUP 26, 29, 30
CULTURAL CONTEXT OF SYMPTOMS 116, 234
CURE
bring miasms to latency 3–4, 206, 212
complete or permanent 2, 3, 13, 185
path to 42, 144, 235–237
CYANOSIS 99, 101–103, 153, 156

D

DAMPNESS AGGRAVATES 118
DANCING
cancer miasm 186, 187, 192
cases with 135, 136, 138, 216, 218
tubercular miasm 151
DANGER, FEELING OF OR ATTRACTION TO 55, 56, 62
DAYTIME AGGRAVATES 20, 21–22, 25, 124, 242
DAYTIME AMELIORATEs 242
DEATH AND DYING 195
DECISIONS, DIFFICULTY MAKING 16, 17
DEFORMITY 65, 76, 239
DENTAL WORK 71–72, 119
DENTITION 21, 25, 26, 123
DEPENDENCE 13, 17, 25
DEPRESSION
case with 196–204
degree evident from interview 161–162
normal in abandoned children 51
sycotic 117
syphilitic 53, 62, 63
DESTRUCTION
syphilitic tendency
mental 55, 58, 63–64
physical 53, 58, 65, 66, 67
tubercular impulse 152, 157
DEVELOPMENTAL ABNORMALITIES 159–160
DEVELOPMENTAL DELAY (CASE) 84–106
DIABETES 124, 190
DIAPER RASH 123, 183
DIARRHEA 6, 22, 25–26, 139, 171
DICTATORIAL NATURE 111, 122, 150, 156
DIGESTION, POOR 20, 23
DIGITALIS 100
DISCHARGES
bloody 65, 67
clear or white 20
gray 65, 67, 68, 72
green or yellow 118, 119, 121, 123
healthy 37, 139, 140, 183
offensive 65
psoric 22
DISCHARGES AGGRAVATE 66
DISEASE
basis of 1–5, 232–233
logic 207
modern 205, 231–232
relation to miasms 67, 143, 184–186, 217
seen through symptoms 9, 105–106
DOGS CHOSEN BY MIASMS 20, 111, 141
DRAFTS OF AIR 22, 28, 137–138
DREAMS 16, 60, 63–64
DROWSINESS 21, 25
DRUG EXPERIENCES 60
DRUG PROBLEMS 65, 149
DRYNESS 21
DULLNESS 53–54, 55–56, 65–66, 76, 221
DUPUYTREN'S DISEASE 70
DYSFUNCTION 66–67

E

EARS
infections of 24–26, 67, 106, 119, 123
psoric dryness of 21
syphilitic deformation of 72
EATING AMELIORATES 21, 23, 28
ECZEMA 27, 124, 128
EGGS, DESIRES 8, 15, 23
EMBARRASSMENT 16, 19
EMOTIONAL SYMPTOMS
cancer 186–189
psora 13–20
sycosis 110–118
syphilis 54–65
tuberculosis 149–153
EMOTIONS, UNEXPRESSED 71, 186, 220
EMPHYSEMA 91, 107
ENCOPRESIS (CASE) 42–52
ENERGY LEVELS 239–240
determine whether miasms are awakened 5–6
high 110, 112, 113
low 13–14, 28

ENLARGEMENTS 118, 120
ENURESIS 29, 39, 45
EPILEPSY 39, 115
ERUPTIONS, SKIN
cases with 133, 209
healthy discharges 27, 184
psoric 21, 25, 28
sycotic 120
EXCESS 111, 118, 120, 239
EXCITEMENT 111–112, 115, 150–152
EXERCISE, MOTIVATIONS FOR 148–149
EXPRESSIVENESS 110, 136
EXTREMES, GOING TO 8, 110, 113
EYES
appearance 153, 154, 155
complaints 23, 67–68, 153, 208

F

FAMILY HISTORY 54, 143, 237
FAMILY MEMBERS, IMPROVEMENT IN ALL 51
FAST MOVEMENT 110, 118, 119
FASTIDIOUSNESS 19, 80, 227
FAT, DESIRE FOR 126, 153, 157
FATIGUE 24, 145
FEAR, AILMENTS FROM 5, 13, 15
FEARFULNESS 13, 25
FEARS
being alone 201
being killed 57
contamination 76
germs 56, 60
killing ones own children 57–58
knives 57
lack of 114, 203
mice 8, 40–41
normal 18, 41, 194
other people, of 55, 56
paralysis 76
psoric 15–16, 18, 27
sycotic 114
FEET, HOT 118, 126, 136, 138
FEVERS
sycotic 118, 119, 135–136, 137
tubercular 145, 153–154, 160, 162, 164–169
FIGHTING 73, 114, 125
FINGERNAILS 19, 23, 82–83, 160, 210
FISHY SMELL 118, 119, 120, 123, 124
FISTULAS 68–69
FIXED IDEAS 32–33, 56
FLUSHING 17, 49, 145, 154
FOUBISTER, DONALD MACDONALD 181–182
FREEDOM, DESIRE FOR 149, 151
FRESH AIR, DESIRE FOR 49, 151–154, 157
FUNCTIONAL DISTURBANCES 20, 23
FUNGUS 82, 83, 169

G

GAMBLING ADDICTIONS 124–125, 126, 131–132
GENITAL PROBLEMS 118, 120–121, 137, 206, 209
GERMS, FEAR OF 56, 60
GONORRHEA
cases with 135, 137, 209
sycotic miasm 109, 121, 124
GOOD IMPRESSION, DESIRE TO MAKE 13, 17, 24–25, 173
GRAY COLORING 65, 66, 68, 72, 202
GREEN DISCHARGES 118, 119, 121, 123
GRIEF
as disease trigger 4–6, 216
psoric 18
sycotic 116–117
syphilitic 61
GROWTH PROBLEMS 25, 29–39, 239
GROWTHS 21, 121
GUILT 13, 16, 18
GUNS 58, 73

H

HAHNEMANN, SAMUEL
on cure 219, 231, 236
on disease 217
miasms, discovery of 1–3
on psora 13
syphilis in his time 53–54
on treating the miasms 109, 144, 179
tuberculosis in his time 144
HAIR LOSS 70, 225
HATRED 58, 61, 63
HAY FEVER 219
HEADACHES 20, 40
HEALTH, RANGE OF NORMALITY FOR 199–200
HEART PROBLEMS 24, 69, 111, 122
HEMORRHOIDS 67, 121
HERING, CONSTANTINE 235–236
HIDING 54, 59, 64, 66, 68

HIGH BLOOD PRESSURE 69, 122, 178
HIV (HUMAN IMMUNODEFICIENCY VIRUS) 205–206, 208–214
HOMEOPATHS AS EXAMPLES 14, 16, 18–19, 22, 114
HYOSCYAMUS 57
HYPERACTIVITY 51–52
HYPERTENSION 69, 122, 178
HYPERTROPHIES 118, 122, 199
HYPOFUNCTIONS 24

I

IDEAS, FIXED 32–33, 56
ILLNESS. *See* Disease
IMPATIENCE 110, 111, 149, 152
IMPRESSIONABILITY 13, 16
IMPROVEMENT, PATIENT. *See also* Cure
- ameliorations and aggravations 236
- danger of 213
- order symptoms are addressed 39–40
- in overall health 10
- ways reported 50

IMPULSIVENESS 110, 114–115, 151, 153, 163
INDEPENDENCE 113–114
INFANTS
- with cancer miasm 181–184
- psoric 25–28, 111
- sycotic 111, 122–123
- syphilitic 72–74
- tubercular 155–156

INFERTILITY 17, 120
INSOMNIA
- carcinosin symptom 181–183, 192
- cases with 78, 80–81, 132
- psoric 20
- sycotic 112–113
- syphilitic 63–64

IRRITABILITY 22, 155
ISOLATING SELF 8, 55, 62
ISOPATHIC THINKING 139, 206–207
ITCHING
- leave alone in children 27
- origin of psora 13
- symptom of psora 17, 21, 25
- symptom of psorinum 28
- symptom of sulphur 8

J

Jealousy 17, 110, 116, 122
JOBS. *See* Professions chosen by miasms

K

KALI BICHROMICUM 211
KALI IODATUM 157
KALI SULPHURICUM 123
KENT, JAMES TYLER 191–192, 219
KIDNEY PROBLEMS 74, 122, 124–134, 170, 190
KILL, URGE TO
- sycotic 115
- syphilitic 55–59, 61, 64

KILLING WITH HOMEOPATHY, UNLIKELINESS OF 104, 194
KNIVES 55, 57, 58–59, 73

L

LACHESIS 100, 232
LANGUAGE OF THE VITAL FORCE, SYMPTOMS AS 9–10, 68, 144
LATENT MIASMS 3–5
LATRODECTUS MACTANS 232
LAUROCERASUS 99–100, 101–104
LEFT-HANDEDNESS 159, 163
LEUCORRHOEA 120
LIGHTNING, LOVE OF 186, 187
LIPS 17–18, 70, 115, 155, 209
LOQUACITY 114, 122, 139, 170
LUNG INFECTIONS 24, 67, 119, 148
LYCOPODIUM 81–82, 104, 128–129, 202, 229

M

MATHEMATICS, INABILITY TO LEARN 55
MEAT, DESIRE FOR 15, 23
MEDORRHINUM
- given in AIDS case 209, 213
- given in MS case 216, 218
- given in sycosis case 128–134, 138, 140
- symptoms 112, 118, 123–124, 140, 156, 199

MENTAL SYMPTOMS
- cancer 186–189
- psora 13–20
- sycosis 110–118
- syphilis 54–65
- tuberculosis 149–153

MERCURIUS 8, 57, 76, 100–101, 163
MERCURY (TREATMENT FOR SYPHILIS) 53
MIASMATIC PRESCRIBING 10–11, 106–108, 231, 237
MIASMS 1–3, 3–5, 143, 205–208
MICE, FEAR OF 8, 40–41
MILK, DESIRE FOR 23, 153, 156, 161

MISERY 55, 62, 63
MODALITIES 242, 244
cancer 189–190
psora 20–25
sycosis 118–122
syphilis 65–72
when to use 194, 237
MODERN POPULATIONS 3, 8, 147, xi
MOLES 181
MOLLUSCA 21
MONONUCLEOSIS 124, 189, 190
MORNING AGGRAVATES 118–119, 242, 244
MORNING AMELIORATES 242
MOUNTAINS, LOVE OF 146, 150–151, 154, 171, 188
MOUTH, TASTES IN 23, 66, 119
MOVEMENT AGGRAVATES 21, 25, 242, 244
MOVEMENT AMELIORATES
sycosis 110, 113, 119, 120, 123
tuberculosis 118, 150, 153
MOVIES 16, 58, 115
MULTIPLE MIASMS
all patients have 9–10, xiii
all remedies have 7–8, xiii
color metaphor 208
difficulty of treating 144, 205
shifting weights of 10–11, 144, 208–214, 218–219, 232–233
MULTIPLE SCLEROSIS (MS) 67, 215–230
MUSCLE ACHES AND CRAMPS 25, 66
MUSCULAR DYSTROPHY **70**
MUSIC, SENSITIVITY TO 150
MUSTY SMELL 118

N

NAILS, POOR 23, 82, 83, 210
NARROW PRESCRIBING 6–7
NATRUM MURIATICUM 31, 189, 222, 223
NATURE, LOVE OF 186, 187, 201
NEPHROTIC SYNDROME 124–134, 190
NERVOUSNESS 19
NEURALGIA 25
NEUROLOGICAL DISEASES 219
NEW SYMPTOMS 1–2
NIGHT AGGRAVATES 15, 65, 76, 242. *See also* Sleep problems
NIGHT AMELIORATES 118, 124, 242
NIGHT SWEATS
psoric 22, 31, 34
tubercular 145, 154, 177
NIGHTLIFE, LOVE OF 110, 112, 124
NITRIC ACID 61
NITRICUM ACIDUM 76
NORMAL, WHAT IS 36, 199–200
NOSODES
of cancer miasm 183, 190
definition 28
psoric 28–29
sycotic 123–124
syphilitic 76
tubercular 156
when to use 11, 185, 192, 207
NUPHAR LUTEUM 202
NUX MOSCHATA 212
NUX VOMICA 15, 41, 175, 177–178

O

OBJECTIVITY IN HOMEOPATHS 18, 19, 35–37, 134, 200
OBSERVATION 19, 202
ODORS. *See* Smells
OLD AGE, TREATING IN 193
OPENNESS 129
OPIUM 99–100, 104
OPTIMISM 145
OSTENTATION 112
OSTEOPOROSIS 23
OUTGOING PERSONALITIES 110
OUTLETS FOR DISTURBANCES, LACK OF 186, 189, 220
OUTSIDE, DESIRE TO BE 49, 99
OVERDOING 110, 117
OVERREACTIONS 114, 239
OVERSENSITIVITY
clairvoyance as 117, 201
psoric 22, 31–32, 48
sycotic 117
tubercular 150
OVERSTIMULATION, MENTAL 113

P

PAIN AS POSITIVE SIGN 224
PAINSTAKING BEHAVIOR 18
PALENESS 17, 154
PAROXYSMS 118, 120
PARTIES, DESIRE FOR 110
PEDUNCULATED GROWTHS 21
PELVIC INFECTIONS 124
PEOPLE, FEAR OF OTHER 55, 56
PERFECTIONISM 186, 188–189, 192, 225

PERMANENT CURES 2, 3, 13, 185
PERSPIRATION 22, 31, 83, 157
PERVERSION 55, 63, 66–67, 239
PHOSPHORUS 100, 128, 155, 157, 202
PIERCING, BODY 63, 115
PLANTAR WARTS 69
PMS (PREMENSTRUAL SYNDROME) 196
POLARITIES, STRONG 110, 117, 124
POLICE OFFICERS 19, 59–60
POSSESSIVENESS 13, 14
POSTPARTUM DEPRESSION 57–58
POTENCIES 34–35, 37–38, 167, 175, 194
POVERTY, FEELING OF 14, 28
POWER 110, 112
PREDISPOSITION 137–138
PREGNANCY 70, 75, 123
PREJUDICE, AVOIDING 19, 35, 200. *See also* Objectivity in homeopaths
PREMENSTRUAL SYNDROME (PMS) 196
PRESCRIBING, MIASMATIC 10–11, 106–108, 231, 237
PROFESSIONS CHOSEN BY MIASMS
  psora 19, 33
  sycosis 112
  syphilis 58–60
  tuberculosis 150
PROGRESSION OF MIASMS 233. *See also* Shifting weight of miasms
PROPORTION, REACTIONS OUT OF 234
PROSTATITIS 120–121, 169–179
PSORA 13–52
  basis of all disease 2–5, 143
  cases with
    cough and delayed growth 29–42
    encopresis and behavior problems 42–52
    marriage problems, depression, anger 200
    multiple sclerosis 227
    nephrotic syndrome 130–131
    prostatitis 174, 178
    reflux and thrush 79
  contrasted to cancer 188
  contrasted to sycosis
    compulsive behavior 118
    energy patterns 113
    fears 114
    fighting 126
    reactions to wind 118
    skin eruptions 120
    warts 121
  contrasted to syphilis
    body piercing 63
    children 73–74
    consolation 72
    dullness 56
    means of spread 54
    school behavior 55
    sexual crimes 64
    violence and killing 58–59
  contrasted to tuberculosis 148
  examples of psoric disease expressions
    asthma 9
    cancer 184
  infant eruptions clear 183
  in infants and children 25–28
  mental and emotional symptoms 13–20
  physical symptoms and modalities 20–25
  remedies 28–29, 28–29
PSORINUM 11, 28–29, 30, 34, 100
PULSATILLA 36

R

RAGE 55, 61
RAPE 17, 64
REACTIONS SHOW THE MIASM 18, 36, 127, 194, 234
REDNESS 8, 17, 119
REFINEMENT 186
REFLUX (CASE) 76–84
RELAPSES 37, 42, 132, 165, 236
REMEDIES
  antidoting 41–42, 41–42
  cancer miasm 190–192
  choosing too early 125
  miasmatic composition of 7–8, xiii
  psoric 28–29
  sycotic 123–124
  syphilitic 75–76
  time they take to work 105
  tubercular 156–157
REPEATING REMEDIES 42, 132–133, 166, 167
REPRODUCTIVE ORGANS, PROBLEMS IN 120–121
RESPIRATORY PROBLEMS 153, 154, 157
REST, BETTER FROM 21
RESTLESSNESS 20
REVENGE 63, 125
RHUS TOXICODENDRON 157
RICH FOOD, DESIRE FOR 23, 126, 146, 153–154, 172–173
RIGIDITY, MENTAL 32–33

RISK-TAKING 112, 113
ROMANTIC FEELINGS AND IDEAS 186
ROTTING 61, 68

S

SACRIFICING 186, 187
SAFETY, DESIRE FOR 13, 20
SALT, DESIRE FOR 154
SANATORIUMS 146
SAVING 13, 14
SCALP, DRY 23
SCHIZOPHRENIA 62
SCIRRHINUM 190
SCLERA, BLUE 153–154, 181, 183, 189–190
SCRATCHING 21, 25, 69
SEA, LOVE OF THE 188, 192, 203
SECRECY 55, 65
SEIZURES 66
SELF-MUTILATION 63
SENSATION, DISTURBANCES OF 23
SENSITIVITY 182–183, 186–187, 192
SENTIMENTALITY 187
SEPIA 100, 103, 170, 189, 202
SEXUAL ABUSE OR CRIMES 17, 64, 127, 216
SEXUAL BEHAVIOR
cases with 171–172, 198
normal 64
psoric 17
spread of sycosis and syphilis 109
sycotic 115–116
syphilitic 64–65
SHIFTING WEIGHT OF MIASMS 10, 144, 208–214, 218–219, 232–233
SHOCK AS DISEASE TRIGGER 4–6, 216
SHOOTING, PRETEND, IN CHILDREN 73, 122
SHYNESS 13, 17, 27, 29, 43
SILENCE 55, 55–56
SILICA 81–83, 155, 157, 227, 229
SIMILLIMUMS 11, 175, 192, 235
SKIN DISEASE, PSORA ORIGINALLY 13
SKIN ERUPTIONS
cases with 133, 209
healthy discharges 27, 184
psoric 21, 25, 28
sycotic 120
SKIN SPOTS, BROWN 118, 120
SLEEP POSITIONS 118, 123, 156
SLEEP PROBLEMS
carcinosin symptom 181–183, 192
cases with 78, 80, 81, 132
psoric 16, 20
sycotic 112–113
syphilitic 63–64
SLOWNESS 13, 22, 24, 28, 239
SMALLNESS 32–33, 182
SMELLS
psoric sour 22, 25
sycotic fishy 118, 119
syphilitic offensive 66, 72
SMOKED FOOD, DESIRE FOR 66, 153, 154, 157
SOUR SMELLS 22, 25
SOUR TASTES, DESIRE FOR 118, 137
SPASMS 118, 120
SPREAD OF MIASMS 2, 54, 109, 143, 206
SRP SYMPTOMS. *See* Strange, rare, peculiar symptoms
STANDING, DIFFICULTY 8, 18, 25
STAPHYSAGRIA 123, 128–129, 186, 222–224
STATE, PRESENT 107–108, 232
STEALING 15, 50
STEROIDS 148
STIFFNESS 120
STOMACH PROBLEMS 20, 24
STOOLS 45–49, 80, 210
STRANGE, RARE, PECULIAR SYMPTOMS
examples of 25, 33, 79–82, 95, 217
how to recognize 35, 234, 237
STRENGTH AND ENDURANCE 110–113
STRESS 5–6, 146
STRIKE, URGE TO 150, 152
STRONG TASTES, DESIRES 118, 119
SUDDEN ONSET 65, 66, 69, 119
SUICIDE 55, 60–61, 74, 96, 117
SULPHUR 7–8, 49–52, 129–130, 140, 189
SUN AGGRAVATES 21–22
SUPPORT, DESIRE FOR 17, 27
SUPPRESSION
awakens miasms 5–7
causes of 6, 70, 77
creates miasms 13, 143, 205
forces energy to find new outlet for symptoms 68–69, 83, 130
SUSCEPTIBILITY 137–138, 147
SUSPICION 55–57, 172, 221
SWEATING 22, 31, 83, 157
SWEETS, DESIRE FOR 21, 49
SWELLING 120, 124, 126, 136, 137
SWINGS, EMOTIONAL 117

SYCOSIS 109–141
cases with
AIDS 209
developmental delay 98
marriage problems, depression, anger 199, 200
MS 216, 217
nephrotic syndrome 124–134
throat infections 134–141
contrasted to psora
love of city 20
reaction to abuse 17
urinary problems 25
contrasted to syphilis
body piercing 63
infants want bouncing 72
contrasted to tuberculosis
energy levels 152
exercising 148
examples of sycotic disease expressions
asthma 9
cancer 184
in infants and children 122–123, 183
mental and emotional symptoms 110–118
physical symptoms and modalities 118–122
remedies 123–124
SYMPTOMS
chasing the 10
choosing which to prescribe on 161–162, 193, 217–218
classifying by miasm 28, 123
cultural context 116
guide to miasms 9–10
language of vital force 68
mental and emotional
cancer 186–189
psora 13–20
sycosis 110–118
syphilis 54–65
tuberculosis 149–153
new 1–2, 236
old returning 37, 177, 194
physical
cancer 189–190
psora 20–25
sycosis 118–122
syphilis 65–72
tuberculosis 153–155
reported only after remedy 105–106
SYPHILINUM 56, 76
SYPHILIS (DISEASE) 53–54, 68, 208–209
SYPHILIS (MIASM) 53–108
cases with
allergies, convulsions, and tantrums 161
developmental delay 84–106
marriage problems, depression, anger 198–199, 200
MS 215
nephrotic syndrome 131
reflux and thrush 76–84
contrasted to cancer 201–202
contrasted to psora
lives apart 20
reaction to abandonment 45
slowness in children 28
contrasted to sycosis
children pretend shooting 122
compulsive behavior 118
fears 114
fighting 125
likes isolation 126
rape 116
sleeplessness 132
warts 121
contrasted to tuberculosis 148
examples of syphilitic disease expressions
asthma 9–10
cancer 184
in infants and children 72–74
mental and emotional symptoms 54–65
physical symptoms and modalities 65–72
remedies 75–76

T

TACHYCARDIA 122
TALKING 18, 114, 122, 137, 139
TANGLED HAIR 23
TANTRUMS 122, 152–153, 155, 158–161
TEETH
grinding 153, 156, 161
point to miasms 71–72
poor 23
present at birth 135, 137, 138
rotting, dreams of 63
TEETHING
fast 123
slow 21, 25, 26
unusual order 74
TEMPERATURES, INTERNAL 22, 66, 118
THROAT INFECTIONS 26, 134–141, 160

THROW, URGE TO 150, 152
THRUSH (CASE) 76–84
THUJA
considered in cases 81, 128–129
given in cases 233
symptoms 121, 123
vaccinations, helps overcome 110
THUNDERSTORMS, LOVE OF 186, 187
TIME TO CURE 219, 235–236
TIMIDITY 17, 18, 25, 27, 29
TOBACCO SMOKE 70–71
TONGUES, CRACKED 72
TONSILLITIS 135, 136
TOUCH SPREADS PSORA 2
TRANQUILIZERS 70
TRAVEL, LOVE OF 150–151, 157, 188, 201, 209
TRAVEL, PREPARATION FOR 14
TREMBLING 19
TRI-MIASMATIC REMEDIES 8, 232
TUBERCULINUM
considered in cases 31, 101, 137
given in cases 163–164, 168, 177
not always for tuberculosis 185
symptoms 156–158
TUBERCULOSIS (DISEASE) 144–145, 146–147
TUBERCULOSIS (MIASM) 143–179
cases with
allergies, convulsions, and tantrums 158–169
developmental delay 98
marriage problems, depression, anger 200
nephrotic syndrome 127–128
prostatitis 169–179
throat infections 135, 138
contrasted to cancer 187
contrasted to sycosis 113
exists only where first three are present 144
in infants and children 155–156
mental and emotional symptoms 149–153
physical symptoms and modalities 153–155
remedies 156–158
TUBERCULOSIS VACCINE 135, 137, 147
TUMORS 121, 189, 190, 191

U

ULCERS 20, 21, 24, 68, 76, 98
UMBILICAL CORD PROBLEMS 74, 94–95, 96, 99
URINARY PROBLEMS 25, 118, 120, 128

V

VACCINATIONS
affect entire organism 53
awaken miasms 109–110, 184
cases with 93, 97, 135, 139
spread miasms 143
suppress vital force 24, 70, 183
thuja helps with 110
VIOLENCE
psoric aversion to 16
syphilitic 54, 57–58, 61, 64–65, 65, 73
tubercular 156
VITAL FORCE OR ENERGY
dETERMINES HOW REMEDIES WORK 39–41, 83
INDIVIDUALIZES DISEASE STATES 215
LEVEL AVAILABLE FOR HEALING 5–6, 193
SYMPTOMS AS ITS LANGUAGE 9–10, 68, 144
WORKs on its own schedule 134, 207
VITILIGO 69
VOMITING (REFLUX CASE) 78, 82, 83

W

WAITING TO PRESCRIBE 106–107, 133–134, 166, 212, 236
WARMTH, BETTER FROM 21, 22
WARTS 21, 69, 109, 121, 123
WASTING 148, 153, 154, 190
WEAKNESS
cancer 183
psora 13–14, 20, 22–24, 29–30, 33–34
tuberculosis 152, 157
WEEPING 36, 46, 49, 72, 124, 234
WEIGHTS OF MULTIPLE MIASMS IN PATIENTS 9–10. *See also* Shifting weight of miasms
WHITE discharges 20, 22
WIND 22, 118, 154
WORRY 13, 16, 19, 24

Y

YELLOW DISCHARGES 118, 119, 121, 123

Made in United States
Orlando, FL
11 November 2026

90609400R00154